MOTIVATION AND WELLBEING FOR STUDENTS

THE PATH TO SUCCESS

BY
FAHIMULLAH
HAYAT

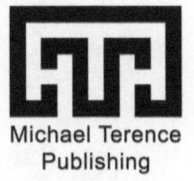

First published in paperback by
Michael Terence Publishing in 2019
www.mtp.agency

Copyright © 2019 Fahimullah Hayat

Fahimullah Hayat has asserted his right to be identified as the
author of this work in accordance with the
Copyright, Designs and Patents Act 1988

ISBN 9781912639694

All rights reserved. No part of this publication may be reproduced, stored
in a retrieval system, or transmitted, in any form or by any means,
electronic, mechanical, photocopying, recording or otherwise, without the
prior permission of the publishers

Edited by
Rahmanullah Hayat and Sadiya Nazmeen Ali

Cover images
Copyright © Chachar

Cover design
Copyright © 2019 Michael Terence Publishing

This book is dedicated to my beautiful family.

I love you all.

MOTIVATION AND WELLBEING FOR STUDENTS

THE PATH TO SUCCESS

BY
FAHIMULLAH
HAYAT

Contents

PART ONE: SELF MOTIVATION 1

Introduction 3

1: Self Motivation and its Importance 5

2: Self Motivation - Building the Techniques 7

3: How to Develop Self Motivation to Beat Shyness 13

4: Self-Improvement Through Positive Self Motivation 17

5: Self Motivation Tips and Strategies 26

6: Two Sides of Self Motivation 37

7: How to Propel Your Career With Self Motivation 40

8: Self-Motivation Finding the Strength to Keep Going 44

PART TWO: TACKLING MENTAL HEALTH ISSUES WHILE RESEARCHING 51

Introduction 53

9: The Power of Mental Health 58

10: Mental Health Issues 63

11: Does Getting Good Sleep Affect Our Ability to Stay Healthy? 118

12: Boost Your Mental Health With The Brain Games!
.... 123

PART THREE: TIME MANAGEMENT 127

13: Learning Time Management Skills 129

14: Time Management Skills - Why They Are Important
.... 131

15: Finishing Your Thesis When You Believe You Can't
.... 158

FINAL NOTE 169

PART ONE: SELF MOTIVATION

Introduction

Self-motivation is imperative. There are a few purposes behind self-motivation which makes it vital in everyone's life. Everyone needs to be self-motivated.

Nowadays, with such vast numbers of challenges out there and a great deal of competition one needs to survive, self-motivation works like a confidence enhancer. It supports ones excitement and gives vitality to work.

Self-motivation is known as the most vital factor in your life. If you are searching for accomplishment in any part of your life, you require self-motivation. Self-motivation is a vital skill to have in order to improve your confidence or self-esteem. It develops a desire to accomplish something great in life. Specialists in the past have accepted and even demonstrated that when self-motivation is joined with self-determination, one can without much of a stretch, move mountains and discover water in deserts.

There are several things one can get motivated with. People get motivated by their strong belief in the almighty. They can even get motivated by the experiences they have had or by any other factor. These things just encourage you to change your perspective in life. One can change into a better person or a better business person with self-motivation.

Let's start with the Vince Lombardi quote:

"Perfection is not attainable, but if we chase perfection we can catch the excellence."

1: Self Motivation and its Importance

People more often than not experience great and tragic occasions in their lives. When thing goes wrong, you have to help yourself, your family and individuals around you. This needs a decent measure of energy reserves within you. While offering help and consolation to your family and companions, you should be extremely strong.

A few people are fortunate to have great help during the times of tribulations. Be that as it may, some are disregarded and require a great deal of courage to endure intense occasions. At such events, one has to get motivated or motivate oneself. The absence of self-motivation at such occasions can be harming and even confound your life further.

Referenced underneath are some solid reasons on why you require self-motivation:

- Self-motivation is critical with regards to accepting difficulties and opportunities in life.
- The power of self-motivation helps in arranging your life and facilitating the difficulties.

- Self-motivation gives another feeling of direction and bearing to your life.
- Self-motivation is vital to give you fulfillment in life.
- Self-motivation gives you a chance to carry on with a satisfying life.
- You can enable and urge yourself to confront extreme occasions and competition in life with the assistance of self-motivation.
- Self-motivation fills you with positive vitality and lifts your energy.
- Self-motivation is essential for your existence. It gives you character and depth.

Motivation is one of the main thrusts that urges a person to go ahead. It is a sort of lift to the fearlessness, confidence and inward inner voice of a man. We all search for some sort of motivation in life. It is relatively difficult to confront an opposition, or make progress to achieve an objective without motivation.

2: Self Motivation - Building the Techniques

Fear and reward are two most commonly utilized strategies to construct motivation in someone. Be that as it may, these strategies are transitory. The main enduring skill is self-motivation. Motivation is the eagerness of accomplishing something. It alludes to inward inclination, powerful urges, and assumption regarding something. You may once in a while free the important dimension of the inner drive to complete something. Self-motivation is the thing that you have, to support the dimension of your internal drive to accomplish your goals.

Self-motivation is a form of self-encouragement. You will state to yourself that you have the ability to improve the situation and in the end get whatever you need in your life. This inward energy will drive you forward until the point of accomplishing your set goals. You may not know about any reward to start with yet you continue chipping away at it. You chip away at it because your inward quality says that you can accomplish your objectives. This is your resolution - the driving force behind your self-motivation. Self-motivation is a combination of willpower, goals, and the ability to continue attaining the highest level of your success.

You need self-motivation to accomplish tasks you have set for yourself. Along the way, you may be faced with situations that are discouraging and can bring down your motivational level. You need to keep yourself really focused on your objectives to maintain the level of your self-motivation. Here are techniques you can adapt to, to start acquiring a higher motivational level and achieve greater success.

Composing Your Plan/Technique

Success does not come easily without a proper plan. Failing to plan is planning to fail. Therefore, you must give a greater emphasis on having a well-prepared plan to achieve your goals. You need to have your plan written on a piece of paper. Having your plan clearly written out gives you a further psychological inner drive, to work toward achieving your goals. You create more enthusiasm and can see more clearly on how you want to achieve your goals. Thus, your commitments will be much stronger.

When recording or writing your goals, state very specific terms, for example, if you want to accumulate a certain amount of money, state exactly how much you want. You must also set a specific date to fulfill your goals and specific rewards for achieving your goals. Writing is not enough if you do not follow up with some reading. You have to make a point to read your written plan at least twice a day, once in the morning before you start your day and one at night just before you go to bed. This simple routine will help you to stay motivated.

Be reasonable, things occur in life. Unanticipated conditions may at times expect you to make modifications in your arrangement. Simply go ahead and make the vital changes. Be that as it may, endeavor to keep up and maintain realistic limits. Try not to make it too simple or too hard for you to accomplish. Set it without flaw to keep up your motivation level.

Picturing Your Goals

You need to simply visualise your goals as much as possible to maintain your motivation at the highest level possible. If your goal is to own an apartment, find pictures of your desired apartment and keep them in front of your eyes. Envisioning your goals makes a positive effect at the forefront of your thoughts and keeps your motivation surging. When you feel exceptionally down, pictures will give the fundamental lift to flood your motivation level positively.

Like the composed plan, you need to make a point to see the visuals something like two times a day. The pictures you see of yourself accomplishing the objectives you want will impart a solid effect in your brain, which will control your daily activities to keep up your dimension of motivation.

Controlling Your Feelings

This one isn't exactly a straightforward activity. It has to do with your inclination in your brain. You have to control what you feel. Your inclination will mirror your psychological mentality and dispositions. If you feel upset and discouraged, you will feel as though everything crashes on you. This inclination considers your physical self. You will lose focus and all that you do will be loaded with mistakes and mishaps along the way. You need to figure out how to begin controlling your inclination.

The easiest way will be to begin your day with a smile. No doubt this can be fake at times due to things that happen around you, but you have got to master this simple task to ensure that things around you will be pleasant and enjoyable for the rest of the day. You can feel the enthusiasm and energy level soaring. You will be able to stay motivated and spread positive energy around you.

Your psychological and physical states of mind work together. Hence, to stay motivated, learn to develop cheerful and confident characters by just walking with your chin up and a smile on your face. You will realize that your confidence and self-motivation levels, are increasing overtime. It is probably kind of hard to maintain the action, but with time, once it naturally becomes your way of life, you can motivate yourself even during difficult times.

Giving Your Effort a Reward

You have to reward yourself for what you have accomplished. This one basically involves being grateful to yourself in accomplishing your goals. You need to credit yourself for what you have experienced, your assurance and your diligent work in guaranteeing your success.

Earlier I said the reward is a temporary method to motivate someone. In this case, a reward is not what keeps you motivated. It is just an element to add flavour to your self-motivation exercise. You may want to think of a simple reward that sounds reasonable with what you have achieved. Do not get over excited about this. Meaning, the reward has to be at par with your level of achievement. Take this positively to enhance your level of self-motivation further.

3: How to Develop Self Motivation to Beat Shyness

Really want to beat shyness? Then it's a stark fact that you're going to need plenty of self-motivation to succeed. Believing in yourself and having self-motivation will lead you towards the life you really want. At its lowest level it's what gets us out of bed in the morning, but when you're full of self-motivation, you really can achieve the life of your dreams.

But, if you're shy or lack confidence, you may well find it hard to get motivated. If this sounds like you, just how can you find self-motivation to beat shyness?
Let us explore a little further...
I'm a firm believer in: "if you want to beat shyness, you'll need to take action". It's self-motivation that forces you to take action.

Chances are if you're shy this will seem very uncomfortable at first. For some shy people, moving outside of their comfort zone can literally make them feel physically sick!

If you don't like pushing yourself and moving outside of your comfort zone then you now have a choice: beat shyness for good so you can enjoy an exciting social life, work towards success, gain more friends and have more romantic encounters, or simply carry on as you are now. That, as I've already mentioned, is the stark reality.

So, you want to beat shyness which is going to take some work and effort on your behalf. And that is why you're going to need plenty of self-motivation. Without it, you're unlikely to succeed.

So, how can we do this?

Motivate yourself to spend half of an hour today to sit down and observe your strengths and weaknesses.

What are you good at? What do you struggle with socially or at work?

This is your first real test of self-motivation. Knowing and understanding the areas you need to work on so you can move forward with confidence and conquer shyness.

You must know yourself before you can get to know

someone else!

Also, thank yourself and appreciate yourself for the things you're good at. This will boost your self-esteem, making you feel more confident. And, confidence overcomes shyness.

So, you must like yourself before you can expect others to like you!

Set yourself small manageable goals.

Obviously, your ultimate goal is to overcome shyness, but it's a step by step process.

Begin with small, simple goals such as making eye contact, smiling and saying "hi" to new people you meet every day.

This will make working towards self-motivation on your part a daily habit, you're going to experience some uncomfortable feelings at first.

Now steely determination must come in. You have to get used to these uncomfortable feelings, it means you're breaking out of your comfort zone and growing mentally stronger.

Put simply:

Self-motivation instills determination and determination brings success!

And for you, success means overcoming shyness, which is your ultimate goal.

Self-motivation will serve you well in life, not just in overcoming shyness, but in everything you do. It will allow you to feel confident in your choices so you can control and live the life you want.

Be the best you can!

4: Self-Improvement Through Positive Self Motivation

Positive Self Motivation is the inward determination that places confidence without hesitation for winning in life. A winner will have the aspiration to improve upon their self development. There never was a consistent winner in any walk of life, who didn't have that burning adopted desire to win. Winners know that the basic developmental axiom in life is the fact that you and I do become what we think about the most. You and I are motivated every day and moved by our currently prevailing thoughts. In other words, we move only in the path of that what we live on, and what we think of.

Everybody in life is self-motivated, a slight bit or a lot it all depends on the person, some negative and some positive. Motivation is a force which causes and move us to act, and it comes from inside of the individuals. Motivation is described as a strong tendency away or toward from a situation or object, and it can be accomplished and developed, it doesn't have to be inborn.

Positive Self Motivation Puts You In The Driver's Seat of Your Life

Anyone willing and hoping to improve upon their personal progress has to, in one way or alternative ignite their motivation. For too long it has been wrongly presumed that motivation is extraneous, that it can be pumped in from the outside through pep talks, or competitions or rallies. Such activities do provide concepts in education, reassurance, and inspiration for individuals to try on their creative powers, but merely if they want to and only if internalized.

That's the secret, and long lasting change is effected only when the need for change is both agreed and internalized. Until the reward or encouragement had been interrupted and internalized it has no motivational power at all. So the real winners in life are the people who have developed, as a result of an complete attitude of positive self-expectancy, a strong positive or self-motivation optimism, This is key to cultivating upon your personal development.

In other words, they developed this capability to change in the direction of their goals that they set for themselves, or roles they want to perform, and they will tolerate anything and make sure nothing distracts them, and they can reach their goals. Despite all the mistakes, discouragement and setbacks, this inner drive continues moving them upward towards their goals and self-fulfillment.

Motivation is an emotional state, and the excessive mental and physical motivators in life, such as, hunger, thirst, survival, love and revenge are all charged with emotion. The two basic emotions which control all human motivation with opposite but nearly the same results are desire and fear.

Fear is the greatest controlling negative motivator of all; fear is the great inhibitor and the excessive compiler, fear tightens, restricts and causes panic, forces and ultimately scuttles plans and makes one feel that they cannot reach their goals anymore. Fear can completely destroy a person's personal growth and constrain any attempt to improve it. Desire equally is like a very strong positive magnet, and it reaches, attracts, opens, and directs, and encourages, and helps to achieve the goals.

Desire and fear are completely apart and opposite to each other, they lead to alternative fates in life, fear continuously looks to the past, and desire looks to the future. Fear vividly replays haunting experiences of failure, pain, unpleasantness and disappointment and is a persistent reminder that the same practices are likely to repeat themselves. The desire on the other hand, triggers a memory of success and pleasure, it excites the need to replay this and to create new winning moments. The consuming prison words of the fearsome person are likely to be, "I have to, I can't, I see risk, and I wish". But desire says, "I want to, I can, I see opportunity, and I will". Desire is that emotional state between where you are and where you would like to be. To have successful personal development, we must learn how to overcome fear alongside desire.

In life, successful people and winners know that all of their actions will be controlled by their thoughts and that you cannot live on the reverse of an idea. That's why you can't stop smoking if you see yourself as a smoker, you can't lose weight if you keep thinking about how fat you are and that's why you can't get rich if you are worried about your bills. Winners see risk as a chance, they see the rewards of success in advance, and they don't see the consequences of failure. They see personal development as a positive step in the direction of a better life. Individuals influenced by fear, they can't act with optimal or positive intent, they go through life reacting in a defensive way. People who are dictated by stress are impotent to change the world they live in, the world they live in adjust them.

It's a sobering and strange, fact that the thing we fear most, we ourselves bring to pass. Scorching desire is the flawless mental anecdote, despair, and for fear. Desire sparks activity which burns up unnecessary adrenaline in the system. It keeps the hope of achievement alive and the mind busy. Successful people in life have strong personal development skills, and they hold a high degree of motivation. The enduring power that moves them to act comes from themselves. Success in life is not reserved for the few, success is almost completely dependent upon persistence and drive.

It is essential to learn and remember how to really develop this winning action quality of positive self-motivation. It's vital for you to remember that everyone is self-motivated, some more so than others, negatively or positively and that motivation is not optional, even the decision to do nonentity task takes some motivation. Each of us is motivated by our desires or fears. Fear is unescapable because it can get you out of danger, and save your life, but as a habit or a way of life, fear has very destructive side-effect.

If we put this into daily life we can that the desire as a green light which allows you to go forward towards your destination and goals, while the fear is like red light which means stop or else you might end up in a crash or points on your licence, so your most valuable exercise in developing positive self-motivation is to try to change and replace fear motivation with desire motivation. Auspiciously, because fear and desire are two sides of the same coin, this is not as hard as it feel like to be. The desire for affluence can replace the fear of poverty.

Good health can replace the fear of sickness, fear of failure can be replaced with a desire for success. All these acts must be existent to improve personal development. A lack of determination is the same as giving-up when there is no real attempt to seek improvement, there can be no improvement at all to relish over. Don't let the fear of failure stop you in your journey for better and bigger personal development, hold onto the desire for complete success and true life gratification. Winners realize that they are motivated by their current thought, so your eyes should be on the return of the success that you pursue, rather than the likely penalty of failure. Make desire your thoughts, and it will drive you with the motivating liveliness for success in every area of your day to day life.

Behind every winner, there is burning desire, of enthusiasm and optimism toward the reward of success and not the penalty of failure, towards the solution in place of the problems and toward the answer in place of the question. Behind every winner there is a burning desire, the must need and the never-ending drive for complete improved personal development.

To Follow are Some Action Reminders Towards Positive Self Motivation!

Most prominently, replace the word "can't" with "can" in the day to day life, you can apply this to nearly 95% of the challenges you come across every day.

Also, replace the word "try" with "will", in your day to day life, this is a method of semantics and establishes your new attitude of living on things you will do rather than on things you plan to try with, that built-in justification in advance for possible failure. Spotlight all your energy and attention on the achievement of the goal you're involved in right now, forget about the consequences of failure. Keep your drive for personal development at the forefront of your mind.

Failure is only a temporary change in a direction to set you straight for your following success. Keep it in mind you usually get what you think of the most. Next, make a list of your five most important desires and wants and right next to each, put down what is the payoffs or benefits is when you complete and achieve it.

Look at the list every morning when you wake up and also every night before you go to sleep. Always give positive feedback to people when they ask you for help and be nice to them. When the problems are your own, focus on the immediate thought... "What's the answer?" Seek out and talk to someone, this week, that is currently doing what it is you want to do most, and be positive that it is someone who is doing it well. This relates to anything, selling or earning, acting, or skiing, speaking, writing, preparing for the exam, managing, or even being a good parent or a partner.

Find an experienced person, get the facts, make a project of learning all you can about other winners in the field. Take a course in it, get personal lessons and generate enthusiasm by mentally long-sighting yourself enjoying the success. Lastly, make it a habit for every one of your goals, to repeat it, and do it again, "I want to, I can, I want to, I can." The power these steps will have on the improvement of your personal development is enormous and not measurable. You will feel permitted, supported, and successful, nothing can stop you, your achievements will pile one upon another, you will know what true personal development feels like in real life, and it is a path to success in your life when you do what you really want you and see the achievements.

5: Self Motivation Tips and Strategies

For some people, self-motivation can be a task in itself. Not every person has the self-control to achieve and reach a job or an assignment without consistent supervision; in any case, in both training and business, it is the most vital piece of the learning proccess. All things considered, past the centre school improvement, an understudy must start the way toward preparing for "this present reality", and part of this procedure incorporates creating self-motivation.

Self-motivation usually starts in school as you figure out how to finish your assignments on time, mainly those that need time outside of the classroom. You can't anticipate that the teacher will be the motivator all the time, so in this manner, you should figure out how to motivate yourself. Without that capacity, your life will be significantly more time-testing since you won't understands how to finish ventures without an irresistible motivation to do as such. At the end of the day, you may clean your home since visitors are coming, yet you won't do it except if something motivates you to do as such because you don't have the foggiest idea about the skill of self-motivation.

The best way to approach the answer to this dilemma is to make a long list of motivation tips. This should include of things that mainly propel you to do things that require to be completed. One thing that encourages numerous individuals is the likelihood that something will come up to keep them from finishing something on time. It doesn't make a difference what it is - school projects, work points of interest, or individual errands - if you find yourself in a situation where you are neglecting to do things currently, may mean you own the powerlessness to do them later, your self-motivation will assume control with the goal that you achieve the assignments in a suitable way.

There is no better motivating factor than facing the possibility that some pre-driven force will prevent you from doing the task if you don't do it right now. For example, if you put off cleaning your house until you expect guests, it opens the possibility of unexpected guests arriving or of something breaking down, and you need to call a repairman. At work, that motivation may be that another more important project arrives on your desk, so now you have two priority projects, and you can't go home until they are completed. There may be other ways, but creating your own stress is one of the best motivation tips that anyone can offer.

Is it accurate to say that you are Self-Motivated?

Is it correct and accurate to say that you are some one who can act certainly motivated with no inconvenience? Or on the other hand, do you battle endeavoring to keep on track and stay focused?

Possibly you discover keeping self-motivated nowadays has turned out to be a greater amount of an upward fight for one of the various reasons. It may be the case that only life, as a rule, has put a huge strain on your motivation capacity so discover approaches to end up self-motivation once more.

Take some time out to review your current situation. Ask yourself where you are going, what goals have you set to accomplish? Reflect where you see yourself and need to be in 5 or 10 years and what estimates you have to set up to arrive. Until the point that you know or can picture your final product, you will battle to act naturally inspired?

So devote time in defining your goals. Write them down carefully, set short and long-term goals for the diverse areas of your life, your own life and professional life. Find out a specific plan you may have, even if it does not fit in with your general life plan. Once your personal and professional goals have been set and recorded this will give you reasons to be self-motivated. Sometimes you could use the career progression development methods by writing your goals on a page alongside how you will achieve them.

Working towards your goals, spending time working on them every day, you will realise and feel your self-motivation at work. You will begin to feel your adrenalin fire you up.

Make sure you do not give up at any time even if you face a challenge and minor setback. Practice in your mind how you would deal with a challenge, and a setback if it happened. Learn how to prepare yourself for this, and if a problem or a delay occurs, you will know how to deal with it and be ready and able to do so.

Occasionally the reason self-motivation is lost is because

you no longer value what you are wanted to achieve then you lose the track or sight of the purpose of being motivated. Maybe your plan has changed, or maybe you have given up on yourself as you don't feel you will be able to achieve what you initially thought you were capable of.

If this is the case, sit down and think about your goals and tell yourself what you are trying to achieve. Should you find your goals have changed, review your plans and set new goals maybe just work on and focus on short-term plans to start with, such as every Friday I will spend an hour to write notes about a class or about a subject or anything you feel like doing but start with something that is easily doable without any problems.

Try not to change and set a new goal every day as it will affect your entire plan, choose a goal that may appear to be the right thing to do, but doesn't feel right to you. Trust your inner feelings on this one.

Become more self-aware of your true feelings, thoughts, and values and be able to understand the goals you reach. As soon as you increase in value the level of your self-awareness, you will be able to realize what your self-motivations are which will help you to achieve greater success in whatever you choose to do.

So when someone asks "are you self-motivated?" you will be able to answer yes in fact I am and if they ask you, "can you do this task alone or without any support?" answer, "yes I can", That is the reason you started and it is your goal, and you will reach it.

Do You Really Need Self Motivation?

You get ready to constitute the last sentence in your "success diary". Looking back over the previous year, you have finished most of your goals. Astounded - you have never felt this effective in your life. You figured out how to lose 10 kgs, take the children to Alton Towers, and how you have completed all the essays, reports and presented your work in conferences, lectures, and many another school, college or university related professions. It had appeared to be an entire deal at the time, however thinking back as you make your last reflection, it appears to be more similar to an undertaking.

Currently, with such achievements close by - you ask

yourself, "Do I really need self-motivation?" You look down at your diary, as it has gone with you all through your past objectives. You understand the time has come to proceed onward to new objectives, and maybe another diary. Be that as it may, will you take self-motivation with you?

Now, it appears as though things in your life have been occurring how you would have preferred them as well, and just as self-motivation was not to credit, in any event not at present. Be that as it may, even with things going your direction, you can at present effectively and rapidly come up short on energy and motivation. What's more, for these occasions, you won't just need your success diary, you may likewise require a little self-improvement.

In this way, as you push ahead onto one year from now's objectives, by following these couple of simple steps, you can keep on keeping your diary close by and remain motivated.

1. **Stay in good company:**

To remain motivated, it is essential and vital to encircle yourself with positive individuals with the end goal to keep a soul of satisfaction alive. Who you invest your energy with will affect your motivation and your fearlessness. Endeavor to consistently connect with "Yes" people. People who remain positive and motivated, never harping on the jobs needing to be done - rather difficult themselves as they advance. If you've seen your current gathering of companions are inadequate here, don't trade them in at this time. Attempt another movement as the week progresses, join a neighbourhood sports alliance, visit with others online or volunteer with a nearby gathering. Pick anything that you are keen on or lifts your spirits, odds are, those individuals are there for a positive social hour and also the movement.

2. **Gain some new useful knowledge:**

Learning is a persistent procedure, which few of us stick to. Each time we gain some new useful knowledge, we feed our motivation since we have expanded our ability and information, keeping our self-confidence level high.

3. **Keep your inspirational state of mind:**

An uplifting state of mind implies a positive personality. Condition yourself to concentrate on the positive qualities in each circumstance, notwithstanding when impediments present themselves. This is a brilliant method to remain on track of self-motivation.

4. **Proceed onward:**

Try not to stall out at the time. It's hard not to fall into negativity, particularly when you're chipping away at a venture or managing issues and, all of a sudden, impediments begin to happen, and you can't advance. At the point when this happens, shift your concentration and approach the circumstance in a different angle. Abruptly, you will see a different disposition and how everything begins to stream the manner in which, you foresaw it too before the obstruction - acknowledging self-motivation has begun to set in by and by.

5. **Write down your feelings:**

You might follow your objectives and ventures in your success diary, yet are you following your inclination also. This is extremely valuable, particularly when you are having episodes of sulkiness. Basically, get your diary, record how you are feeling - and the reason you're feeling the manner in which you are. Do likewise, notwithstanding when you are feeling sheer satisfaction. This will enable you to perceive any examples through your diary chronicles, which will assist you with deciphering your feelings - what brings you misery and what brings you joy.

6. **Keep tabs on your development:**

Alright, I realize you're as of now doing this with your diary. In any case, did you realize that we, for the most part, measure our victories and not simply the occasions we feel self-motivation? Utilize your diary to record these minutes too. Additionally, on days when you are feeling low, browse through your advancement to be helped to remember your achievements, and rapidly begin feeling better once more, as you proceed with the cycle of the finishing of an objective.

7. **Start sharing:**

Not only is sharing something worth doing, but it's also additionally a beyond any doubt shot approach to get motivated. When you realize you could contribute even in the smallest way that is available, you will feel motivated to improve the situation. Sharing ideas, thoughts, and feelings, or notwithstanding motivating a companion who are feeling low, will rapidly expand your self-assurance.

Keeping up self-motivation isn't in every case, simple. Be that as it may, as you adventure towards your objectives, recall all voyages start with an initial step. So why not take yours today?

6: Two Sides of Self Motivation

Self-motivation can be divided into two perspectives. The first is oneself motivation whence of the exercises that are associated with the behavior. Also, the other one is when people are motivated as a result of the expression of remuneration when something is determined.

These two sorts of self-motivation are called intrinsic and extrinsic self-motivation.

Extrinsic self-motivation: This kind of self-motivation can be seen unmistakably in the workhouse. A portion of the people who are raveled may not be experts in the field, but rather they keep on being a part of the group, for of the offer of high pay and rewards given them.

The prizes are not just in the position of cash. It can be in the form of, identification or status and so on. You realize that if you work sufficiently, you can be placed in a more noteworthy position and will rise to acquire the sort of cash you generally wanted. That is the self-motivation that makes you go to work as the day progressed.

With, the competition that is taking place in companies widespread, it is not that easy anymore for a person to concentrate on motivation. Companies are gradual increasing the compensation and rewards that they present to keep up with what others are acting on. Most of the duration employees are not enticed by these rewards anymore. This is because they decide that they can have them with some other company. This is the downside of extraneous self-motivation. You can never tell how far you would go, for another person to remain motivated.

Intrinsic self-motivation: This is the sort of self-motivation where activities are completed with no another exterior factors involved. This basically means that some one likes what he is doing and is not coaxed into it just after all there is a word of a reward later on. It can be recognized that intrinsic self motivation is the reason why personal growth was achieved by those in their early stages of existence.

How do you conceive that you are experiencing intrinsic self-motivation? It is when you possess those deep thoughts within you, you have the potential of achieving the world you want for so long. It can be because you have this necessary innate strength within you. Without the obligation of anything, you want to get into the doing to be able to self-train your strength.

Secondly, you want to set an example and stand out to others that they too can do it. Considering it is the force and the ability that is pushing a person to reach for his personal goals, it cannot be blamed on minimum chances or the perfect chance, as to why you are there. It is because you decide and you can. Lastly is when you want to turn into an authority in the arena that you love doing. It will all depend upon your selection and the truth that you love what you do. Becoming an authority in the field is the main affair on your intellect.

Whatsoever sort of self-motivation it is, the main intention is to reach for the personal goals you have set for yourself. It does not matter what self-motivation method you are on, what matters is for you to project to your self to turn out successful.

7: How to Propel Your Career With Self Motivation

Have you at any point thought about how effective people utilize self-motivation to propel their careers? It's no secret that motivated people advance quicker, further and earn more than less motivated people. But you can't just say you are motivated to do more and expect instant success. You've got to believe in self-motivation and practice the habits to realize maximum achievement.

Many of us find ourselves trapped in a dead-end job with a lack of direction. "I just don't know what I want to do", "Nothing is working for me". Your life is plain and boring, yet deep down you want more out of life.

You can find examples of success all around you. Regardless of your interests or career path, you want to pursue, you can find people everywhere who have succeeded. The 'secret' is that our seeds to success are right in front of us-- it's hidden in plain sight, and those individuals who have learned self-motivation techniques unlock those hidden features to move forward and create success.

Ask yourself for a moment, how is it that some people face adversity and are able to break away quickly and accomplish great things while others sit and watch on the sidelines. It's never the situation but the outcome that determines our success. It takes focus, determination and above all, action to succeed. I often see the same people everyday spending, so much time wishing they could and wanting to move forward but just find it difficult to change direction.

Self-motivation gives you this overwhelming inspiration to perform a radical shift; it's like your own kick-start every day to move from ordinary to extraordinary. You know that "new year" resolution feeling you get to start anew and make things happen? Well, self-motivation helps you tap into your inner energy and promote those objectives and remain focused to actually achieve them, instead of just thinking and talking about them.

As insane as it may sound, many of us are like zombies, just there taking up space. We think, but don't act. We watch, but never really see what is going on. We question but have little idea how to arrive at our goal. What if all of a sudden you could find direction? That critical piece of the puzzle that would translate everything into strength and passion?

Just imagine for a moment writing down a list of goals that you want and need to accomplish within a short period. What's more, imagine writing down in detail how to accomplish every goal on your list than starting your day actually striving to achieve it. Can you do this? Of course, you can. All you need is a self-motivating attitude that kick-starts your day on a positive footing.

Take some time and watch the people around you. Unmotivated people seem bored, lack enthusiasm and irritable all the time. They never notice any of life's rewards and seem to always focus on the negative. Strategies in self-motivation will teach you how to move forward in spite of the insurmountable obstacles you may be faced with.

When you increase your motivation and learn how to hone it, you become inspired to live up to your full potential. You excel and enjoy life, and truly see things differently. Most importantly, you start to realize the benefits and everything that's available to you.

Many people still don't realize what's really out there; they've never been inspired to look further than where they are right now. They dream about living an awesome life but reject the idea because they're not motivated to believe in themselves. By investing a small amount of effort in motivating yourself, you can improve every area of your life.

8: Self-Motivation Finding the Strength to Keep Going

Discover The Strength To Keep Going

With regards to self-motivation, one thing you need to recall isn't surrendering when things are extraordinary. You don't have time for that. When you get to the best and when you feel the best, an accomplishment in any aspects of your life, you at long last have the decent car or that great job, you can in the end, begin getting lazy.

Keep in mind a certain thing; you can't be wasting your time doing that. You need to do all that you can to not lose your strategy, your self-motivation; and above all dependably keep that deep longing splendid constantly.

You don't have time to loosen up, or you'll fail.

You can't stop!

One thing you need to continually remind yourself is you can't stop regardless. It doesn't make a difference how great and successful you will be; you can't quit dealing with yourself. This is your golden rule to live by.

Even when you believe that you don't have any room for self-improvement you need more of it; there is room for getting better and stronger.

Self-motivation is continually taking a shot at you. There's dependably room; there will dependably be more space for you. You are not born into the world as perfection and you never will be perfection. So you will always need to continue working on yourself.

You need to continue taking a shot at yourself; it's the main way. Try not to trick yourself that you're finished, just because you accomplished your objective. Oh no, no, no, no!

There is a whole other world to you that you can enhance and should meet. You dove into this self-motivation journey for a particular reason. You need the best for you and your family. This is a procedure that will request the most out of you.

You have picked this life. There is no time for resting quite recently. You should work, ready your leafy foods and attend to the desserts later.

Try not to Play Around

What I need you to get from this is you have no space to loosen up or get lazy. That isn't you. This thought should never run over your brain. You are superior to this. You're a man that is on a consistent adventure for self-motivation, personal development whatever it is youre working for.

You are a man who accepts and merits more, merits better and needs to live more noteworthy. The main way you'll improve is by being as well as can be expected to be all around, by always taking a shot at your self.

As you continue developing in life remind yourself what you're going for; what it is that you're shooting for? This will enable you to continue developing in life and improving as a man in life.

I am revealing this to you since I have seen effective people and when they meet their goals they effortlessly free up. Some have even lost everything in light of the fact that they have quit doing what they should do.

They quit making improvements to their bodies, their brain, and their career. They felt it was alright to stop what they were doing that got them there in the first place. Arrogance is fatal. You must be cautious with that.

They lost all that they have worked for notwithstanding when you trust that you don't have to continue to keep working on yourself despite everything you have space to work on yourself more.

You are brighter than you are, trust yourself and continue working on yourself. Try not to stop.

Keep yourself sound, stable, and above all watchful consistently because you will slip and fall and lose all that you have worked for.

You need to secure your dream, your wants, and desires, shield yourself from when you're feeling down. You don't want to fall down back to the start of your journey on self-motivation.

Help yourself arrive to this point. If nobody else can enable you to arrive quicker at that point make an arrangement, maintain it and keep it alongside you without stopping for even a minute.

Have your plan under your pillow and sleep on it so you can remind yourself that you have to keep working on yourself every day even when you're successful.

I know it's tiring, but you have to do it. You want to be successful, don't you? This is part of you, doing habits, creating rituals, it's your daily diet.

You need to take a gander at your arrangement and work on it and work on it as though your life depended upon it.

Whatever it is that you want most in life whether that be a job, material ownership, riches, a family; you can't manage the cost of slacking off quickly. This isn't you and doesn't begin now.

Continuously, I mean this, dependably continue working on yourself until the point when you turn out to be so damn incredible that keeping up yourself at that dimension turns out to be simple.

The main adversary you will confront is yourself with regards to consistent self-motivation. You need to continue battling with yourself regularly and once you overcome yourself, you will have another you.

Nobody is your enemy, except yourself. Overcome your frightened self, and you'll win in the game called life.

How solid you get how keen you get depends all entirely to you. Figure out how to be solid, figure out how to be careful, when you see yourself slacking off.

Try not to give your negative voice a chance to win, you are here in this world to carry on with a superior life you merit, and you have to go get it.

Life won't stroll up to you at your front door and hand it to you, except if you're brought into the world an extremely rich person however that isn't you. Work for your dreams, work for your desires, you have to work on yourself first. You first, desires second.

To wrap things up, do every one of these things above and you'll accomplish self-mastery of yourself, and nothing on the planet will stop you. You'll turn into a lot more of a joyful person, peaceful and self-inspired and self-motivated.

PART TWO: TACKLING MENTAL HEALTH ISSUES WHILE RESEARCHING

Introduction

Researching in your dream field should be the adventure of a lifetime.

That's why it can be so disappointing when your mental health, while studying abroad gets in the way of you completing your thesis on time.

These symptoms of culture shock could last anywhere from a few days to a few weeks. This is completely normal for a finishing research experience. The key to tackling these issues is just to push through — immerse yourself in the culture, get to know where the issue is coming from, push-through and at the end of the day, you will come out victorious.

It will get easier every time you go outside if you're actively learning to deal with it. It's not normal, however, to experience these symptoms longer than a month or two. If you do, you might be developing some form of depression or anxiety. And there's a good chance that many of us will experience this first hand, as recent figures suggest that one in four of us will experience mental health issues while researching. Given there remains a stigma about talking about this, these figures could still be vastly underrepresented.

Grad students are at risk of having trouble with their mental health. These triggers can come in many forms; stress, bullying, losing a loved one, feeling isolated from family or friends, a family break up or divorce, financial strain, problems with physical health, toxic relationships, lifestyle changes (e.g. the birth of a child) to a feeling of being overwhelmed with having too much to cope with on a day to day basis. The list is endless. Most of us will be affected by at least one of these things in our lives, so why does mental health remain stigmatized, and a discussion that needs to stay behind closed doors?

In recent years awareness and understanding of mental health is definitely on the increase, thanks to the rise in public figures discussing their experiences with mental health (Prince William and Harry's recent documentary and support of Minds Together showed people that anyone could struggle to manage their Mental Health effectively) irrespective of status or your financial situation. Alongside this, there have been the devastating stories of those that do not come through it, like Robin Williams taking his life after his battle with depression. The brave people who talk about it publically help to raise awareness and help to remove the stigma that surrounds it, but the battle won't be won until mental health is taken as seriously as physical health.

Say you break your leg, what do you do? The answer is simple... you go to see a doctor. But if you start to struggle with anxiety or depression, what do you do? The answer is much more complex. The reality is many sit there and struggle, trying to work out why they feel the way they do, and questioning themselves on whether there is really something wrong with them. The idea of even talking about it with someone makes them freeze. Even if they do consider the doctor, they often question whether they will be taken seriously. So, before we even deal with waiting lists (often months!) for treatment, there's a number of challenges to overcome.

We acknowledge understanding and support for mental health has come a long way but we have only scratched the surface, and there's still a very long journey ahead. I do believe that a core factor in managing this health condition is through breaking down the social barriers and growing knowledge and understanding of not only the topic itsel,f but also the additional challenges people may be facing. A deep exploration of context is crucial to understanding, and something we build into all of our research studies.

Different independent organizations have tackled this from a number of angles; whether it's the impact of debt and money concerns, the interrelationship of drugs and mental health, helping young people build resilience, and how to spot the early signs in friends through their social media posts.

Building blocks of happiness and how these can help young people protect themselves from what life can throw at them along the way has also been looked into over the years.

In our society, today, going about in our daily routine can be stressful enough, but trying to juggle family or a job with researching while experiencing mental illness can make it that much harder. But students can work through many challenges and still perform well and achieve their respective goals. In this very part of this book, I will give details on tackling mental health issues while researching.

Firstly, I will dive right into Mental Health in general and at the later part, I will focus on tackling mental health while researching, how you can finish up your thesis when you believe you can't.

"You, yourself, as much as anybody in the entire universe, deserve your love and affection" – The Buddha.

9: The Power of Mental Health

Mental health is something every student wants for themselves, whether we know it by name or not. There are no easy answers here - mental fitness is the awkward stepchild you sent away to the state hospital in the country and visited once a year.

In fact, good mental health is an integral part of good overall health for people with HIV. Primary Care Mental Condition is a new, peer-reviewed journal on research, education, development, and delivery of mental health in primary care. But mental health is far more than merely the absence of mental illness.

Depressions are the greatest Problem

People are four times more likely to break off a romantic relationship if their partner is diagnosed with severe depression than if they develop a physical disability. Overall, the two strongest predictors for thinking about suicide were depression and substance abuse.

Through compelling personal stories told through; television, video, the Internet, and print media, the campaign encourages men to recognize depression and its impact on their; work, home, and community life. However, it will also enable Cam-mind to launch a project designed to help employers tackle; stress, anxiety, and depression in the workplace. But what's the difference between "normal" feelings of sadness and the feelings caused by depression.

Topics covered vary widely, from healthy self-esteem in adolescence and signs of depression to resources for diagnosing mental health problems in children.

Problems about Mental Condition

Those with schizophrenia are particularly likely to face problems: 20% of women said they would break up with a partner who was diagnosed with the condition. The research team have also found that stress at work is associated with a 50 percent excess risk of coronary heart disease, and there is consistent evidence that jobs with high demands, low control, and effort-reward imbalance are risk factors for mental and physical health problems (major depression, anxiety disorders, and substance use disorders).

The Mental Condition and Poverty Project called on the SAHRC to consider setting up a commission that will primarily focus on the needs of people with mental health problems. Even the best-trained psychiatrists do not necessarily have an internship in the problems of normal living. What many people don't realize is that we all have mental health - just as we have physical health - and that mental health problems can affect anyone, whatever their age or background.

Psychological therapies are based on talking and working with people to understand the causes and triggers of mental health problems and developing practical strategies to deal with them.

Searching for Information

The first step is to reduce the stigma surrounding mental

illnesses, using targeted public education activities that are designed to provide the public with factual information about mental illnesses and to suggest strategies for enhancing mental fitness, much like anti-smoking campaigns promote physical health.

It, therefore, makes good sense for people with HIV to have information about the ways in which HIV can affect their mental health and about common mental fitness issues such as depression, anxiety, and emotional distress. This comprehensive information resource for child mental Condition and parenting information includes articles; resources, a glossary, and Ask the Expert section, a disorder guide, publications, and FAQs.

These offer useful information explaining educational evaluations, and also lists interventions that may be used to address various mental fitness conditions, including; anxiety, obsessive-compulsive disorder, depression, bipolar disorder, ADHD, autism spectrum disorders, and more.

Mental Condition is more important than physical health. Mental fitness is more than the absence of mental disorders. Mental health can be conceptualized as a state of well-being in which the individual realizes his or her abilities, can cope with the normal stresses of life, can work productively and fruitfully, and is able to make a contribution to his or her community.

In this positive sense, mental health is the foundation for well-being and effective functioning for an individual and a community.

10: Mental Health Issues

The American College Health Association (ACHA) reports that any number of factors — chronic pain, allergies, gaming, excessive Internet use, relationship problems, gambling — can affect us day in day out, these may affect our performances in work or academic performance for students. However, psychiatrically or medically diagnosed challenges such as stress, anxiety, and depression generally have a greater impact and may require a more thoughtful approach to guidance or treatment.

In the next few chapters, I will dive into more specific information about a variety of common mental health challenges and focus on where and how we can turn to for support.

Stress and Anxiety

What are stress and anxiety?

Most people experience stress and anxiety from time to time. Stress is any demand placed on your brain or physical body. People can report feeling stressed when multiple competing demands are placed on them. The feeling of being stressed can be triggered by an event that makes you feel frustrated or nervous. Anxiety is a feeling of fear, worry, or unease. It can be a reaction to stress, or it can occur in people who are unable to identify significant stressors in their life.

Stress and anxiety are not always bad. In the short term, they can help you overcome a challenge or a dangerous situation. Examples of everyday stress and anxiety include worrying about finding a job, feeling nervous before a big test, or being embarrassed in certain social situations. If we did not experience some anxiety, we might not be motivated to do things that we need to do (for instance, studying for that big test!).

However, if stress and anxiety begin interfering with your daily life, and it may indicate a more serious issue. If you are avoiding situations due to irrational fears, constantly worrying, or experiencing severe anxiety about a traumatic event weeks after it happened, it may be time to seek help.

What does stress and anxiety feel like?

Stress and anxiety can produce both physical and psychological symptoms. People experience stress and anxiety differently. Common physical symptoms include:

- Stomach ache
- Muscle tension
- Headache
- Rapid breathing
- Fast heartbeat
- Sweating
- Shaking
- Dizziness
- Frequent urination
- Change in appetite
- Trouble sleeping
- Diarrhea
- Fatigue

Stress and anxiety can cause mental or emotional symptoms in addition to physical ones. These can include:

- Feelings of impending doom
- Panic or nervousness, especially in social settings
- Difficulty concentrating
- Irrational anger
- Restlessness

People who have stress and anxiety over long periods may experience negative related health outcomes. They are more likely to develop heart disease, high blood pressure, diabetes, and may even develop depression and panic disorder.

What causes stress and anxiety?

For most people, stress, and anxiety come and go. They usually occur after particular life events, but then go away.

Common Causes

Common stressors include:

- Moving

- Starting a new school or job
- Having an illness or injury
- Having a friend or family member who is ill or injured
- Death of a family member or friend
- Getting married
- Having a baby

Drugs and medications

Drugs that contain stimulants may make the symptoms of stress and anxiety worse. Regular use of caffeine, illicit drugs such as cocaine, and even alcohol can also make symptoms worse.

Prescription medications that can make symptoms worse include:

- Thyroid medications
- Asthma inhalers
- Diet pills

Stress- and anxiety-related disorders

Stress and anxiety that occurs frequently or seems out of

proportion to the stressor may be signs of an anxiety disorder. An estimated 40 million Americans live with some type of anxiety disorder.

People with these disorders may feel anxious and stressed on a daily basis and for prolonged periods of time. These disorders include the following:

• Generalized anxiety disorder (GAD) is a common anxiety disorder characterized by uncontrollable worrying. Sometimes people worry about bad things happening to them or their loved ones, and at other times they may not be able to identify any source of worry.

• Panic disorder is a condition that causes panic attacks, which are moments of extreme fear accompanied by a pounding heart, shortness of breath, and a fear of impending doom.

• Post-traumatic stress disorder (PTSD) is a condition that causes flashbacks or anxiety as a result of a traumatic experience. I will go into details about PTSD in a later chapter of this book.

• Social phobia is a condition that causes intense feelings

of anxiety in situations that involve interacting with others.

• Obsessive-compulsive disorder is a condition that causes repetitive thoughts and the compulsion to complete certain ritual actions.

When to seek help

If you're having thoughts about harming yourself or others, you should seek immediate medical help. Stress and anxiety are treatable conditions, and there are many resources, strategies, and treatments that can help. If you're unable to control your worries, and stress is impacting your daily life, talk to your primary care provider about ways to manage stress and anxiety.

Techniques to manage stress and anxiety

It's normal to experience stress and anxiety from time to time, and there are strategies you can use to make them more manageable. Pay attention to how your body and mind respond to stressful and anxiety-producing situations. Next time a stressful experience occurs, you'll be able to anticipate your reaction, and it may be less disruptive.

Managing everyday stress and anxiety

Certain lifestyle changes can help alleviate symptoms of stress and anxiety. These techniques can be used along with medical treatments for anxiety. Techniques to reduce stress and anxiety include:

- Eating a balanced, healthy diet
- Limiting caffeine and alcohol consumption
- Getting enough sleep
- Getting regular exercise
- Meditating
- Scheduling time for hobbies
- Keeping a diary of your feelings
- Practicing deep breathing
- Recognizing the factors that trigger your stress
- Talking to a friend

Be mindful if you tend to use substances like alcohol or

drugs as ways to cope with stress and anxiety. This can lead to serious substance abuse issues that can make stress and anxiety worse.

Seeking professional help for stress and anxiety

There are many ways to seek treatment for stress and anxiety. If you feel like you're unable to cope with stress and anxiety, your primary care provider may suggest that you see a mental health provider. They may use psychotherapy, also known as talk therapy, to help you work through your stress and anxiety. Your therapist may also teach you applied relaxation techniques to help you manage stress.

Cognitive behavioral therapy (CBT) is a popular and effective method used to manage anxiety. This type of therapy teaches you to recognize anxious thoughts and behaviors and change them into more positive ones.

Exposure therapy and systematic desensitization can be effective in treating phobias. They involve gradually exposing you to anxiety-provoking stimuli to help manage your feelings of fear.

Medications

Your primary care provider may also recommend medication to help treat a diagnosed anxiety disorder. These may include selective-serotonin reuptake inhibitors (SSRIs) such as sertraline (Zoloft) or paroxetine (Paxil). Sometimes providers use anti-anxiety medications (benzodiazepines), such as diazepam (Valium) or lorazepam (Ativan), but these approaches are generally used on a short-term basis due to the risk of addiction.

What is the long-term outlook for stress and anxiety?

Stress and anxiety can be unpleasant to deal with. They can also have negative effects on your physical health if untreated for long periods. While some amount of stress and anxiety in life is expected and shouldn't be cause for concern, it's important to recognize when the stress in your life is causing negative consequences. If you feel like your stress and anxiety are becoming unmanageable, seek professional help or ask others to help you find the support you need.

Depression

Depression is one of the most common mental illnesses affecting many people across the world

It is a common and a serious mental illness in which feelings of sadness, loss of interest, angry, frustration, or other negative emotions like irritability (especially in adolescents). Depression could last for weeks to months and to years, it affects individual day to day life.

As humans we all feel stressed and have bad days in school, colleges and university usually we refer to them as feeling sad or blue, but these feeling generally pass in few days and no sign of depressions.

As we know depression can cause deep emotional pain both to the person experiencing depression and, usually people around the person, who is affected such as family and close friends or could affect colleagues.

Depression is a major public-health issue. It is the

foremost cause of disability in for people between ages 15 and 44 and is the number one cause of injury or illness for men and women around the globe. People with depression is more likely to die from suicide as well as from other illnesses, such as heart disease.

What Is Depression?

There are numerous different types of medically recognized depression.

The furthermost common type of depression is called major depression, and it happens when symptoms interfere with the day to day activities of life or with daily functions — including, reading a book, attending class, work, getting ready for the exam, sleep, and eating habits. In the mildest form depression can be feeling low, sad or make you feel like doing nothing but then the most severe depression can be life-threatening because it could lead one feeling suicidal or they give up on everything and everything.

If we compare how people differ from depression it could

be very different from person to person, sometimes people suffer or experience significant depression at a point in their life, while some other people may go through many occasions of major depressions and reoccurrence of the same problem lead to serve depression.

In contrast, people with a condition known as a persistent depressive disorder — also identified as dysthymia — experience a depressed mood that lasts continuously for few years

Other familiar types of depression include:

• **Postpartum depression**, it causes mothers to experience symptoms of serve depression after giving birth. In this case, the mood impairment is extreme and lasts for a long time. The symptoms of this could be feeling extreme sadness, anxious or exhaustion can make it difficult for the mother to bond with the baby.

• **Seasonal affective disorder,** this is caused by the lack of sunlight it usually occurs during winter time and sometimes in spring- in the UK it will be more likely in around end of October to end of March as that's when the days are so short, and it is mostly dark outside. This depression is usually coming by social withdrawal and lots of sleep and mostly weight gain.

• **Major depression with psychotic features**, this is the severe type of depression which causes hearing or seeing things other people can't hear or see.

How Many People Experience Depression?

As we can see from the definition that depression is feeling low, sad or just feel like doing nothing which suggests that someone at some point in their life, will be suffering from depression and it is the most common mental health disorder. Depression is becoming more prevalent, especially among adolescents.

According to the everyday health website, In 2016, 16.2 million adults age 18 older — almost 6.7 per cent of adults — had at least one major depressive episode. Additionally, 3.1 million adolescents — 19.4 percent of girls and 6.4 per cent of boys — have experienced major depression. The increase in depression rates among adolescents has outpaced all other age groups.

Persistent depressive disorder affects about 1.5 percent of the adult population.

According to the NIH, women in the U.S. are significantly more likely to experience depression (8.5 percent) than men (4.8 percent).

Among adults, people between ages 18 and 25 are most at risk for depression (10.9 percent), whereas those older than the age of 50 are at the lowest risk (4.8 percent).

When racial and ethnic factors are considered, adults who identify with two or more racial or ethnic groups show the highest rate of depression (10.5 percent).

Having one depressive episode increases your risk of having another later in life. According to a study in Psychological Medicine, more than 13 percent of people who recover from their first episode of major depression go on to have another episode within five years; 23 percent within ten years; and 42 percent within 20 years.

According to the World Health Organization (WHO). globally, depression affects more than 300 million people of all ages, That is the corresponding of 4.4 percent of the global population.

Depression is the main cause of disability globally. Fewer than half of those living with depression — and in some countries, fewer than 10 percent, seek the care they need. Some factors prevent people from getting treatment, such as misdiagnosis, lack of trained healthcare professionals to detect the mental health and social stigma.

What Causes Depression?

There are many different reasons which could trigger the on-start of depression, including grief, being long-term ill chronic pain, cancer, diabetes or any other long-term diseases, stressful life events such as going through a divorce, losing a job. Depression could also start all of sudden spontaneously, without any understandable cause.

A person who experiences anxiety is at high risk for emerging depression, and vice versa. People that are diagnosed with anxiety could be developing or already developed and diagnosed with depression.

Researchers are not sure exactly why some people

develop depression and others evade it. Many factors most likely contribute to the development of depression, including:

• Genetics and Biology, it is a mood disorder, and suicide within a family history can increase the percentage possibility of a family member attempting suicide.

• Trauma or abuse at an early age, can cause long-term changes in how the brain reacts with stress and fear.

• Brain structure and chemistry imbalance, research shows that depression causes imbalance in neurotransmitters which is involved in mood regulation. Further studies have revealed that the frontal lobe becomes less active when a person is depressed.

• Substance abuse, most of the time people who abuse drugs or alcohol also have depression, requiring a coordinated treatment approach.

• Other medical conditions, people with a long-term illness such as cancer, sleep disorders and chronic pain are further expected to develop depression.

How Can You Tell if You Are Depressed?

Everyone has times when they feel extremely sad and frustrated, or can't be bothered to do anything kind of feeling. But unless your life is conquered by negative feelings on most days, for most of the day, for weeks on end, you may not have depression.

It is extremely difficult to understand all the complicated ways that depression can occur- in women, men and increasingly in teenagers—is the first step towards finding the correct treatment for mental health illness, as World Health Organisation (WHO) estimated 300 million people around the world suffer from depression, which would mean all 300 million people would differ within symptoms of depression and the type of depression they have, and therefore treatment would be difficult to generalise to all those that suffer from depression

Depression symptoms can vary from person to person, and depend on an individuals age and sex. Usually, adults with depression can be very sad. Women with depression are more likely to be anxious and indecisive, while men are more likely to react with aggression and anger.

If you think, you may have depression, seek medical help. If you are a school, college or university student speak with your mental health and wellbeing teams, they will be able to direct you to the right place.

At the end of the book, I will share a list of websites and resources which could be used by anyone in the UK and around the world to seek help and information.

What Are the Treatment Options for Depression?

The vast majority of people with depression who seek treatment will find a cure, with success rates of about 80 or 90 percent. But getting treatment it isn't easy. Finding the right approach and treatment can be a long process of trial and error, as the options expand and become more targeted to each patient's particular needs.

For people looking for medication-free help, there are more choices than ever — from acupuncture, meditation, and yoga to cognitive behavioral therapy, designed to replace harmful patterns in one's thoughts with healthy ones.

Antidepressants remain a powerful tool, especially as researchers learn more about brain chemistry and develop new drugs that better neurological imbalances, with fewer side effects.

For the most intractable cases of depression, physicians may turn to brain-stimulation treatments like electroconvulsive therapy (ECT). ECT can provide fast relief with far fewer side effects than electroshock therapy did so infamously.

At the other end of the spectrum, researchers are exploring a salvage medication for people with suicidal depression: ketamine is a controlled class B drug, under the misuse of drugs act 1971. It is a street drug that can induce hallucinations and out-of-body experiences but has been thought to provide relief from depression. Ketamine is currently undergoing clinical trials; meanwhile, physicians warn that this drug can be abused.

Will Medication Work Against Depression?

When lifestyle changes or psychotherapy aren't lifting the

pall of depression, antidepressants typically come into play. An estimated 13 percent of Americans age 12 and above take antidepressants — a 65 percent increase from 1999 to 2014.

Understanding the main pharmaceutical options requires becoming familiar with a number of acronyms: SSRIs (selective serotonin reuptake inhibitors), SNRIs (serotonin and norepinephrine reuptake inhibitors), NDRIs (norepinephrine–dopamine reuptake inhibitors), TCAs (tricyclic antidepressants), and MAOIs (monoamine oxidase inhibitors). These represent categories of drugs, grouped together because of their effect on various neurotransmitters (chemical messengers) in the brain.

SSRIs (selective serotonin reuptake inhibitors) like Prozac (fluoxetine), Celexa (citalopram), and Zoloft (sertraline) are the most commonly prescribed antidepressants. They target serotonin, a neurotransmitter that helps control mood, appetite, and sleep. People with depression often have abnormally low levels of serotonin.

All antidepressants can have side effects, but some may be more problematic than others. Guided by your doctor, you may need to try several different drugs before you find the one that's best for you. Keep in mind that they do not work immediately and usually take at least several weeks for maximal benefit. Combining the right medication with psychotherapy or another intervention, like a support group, might be what you need, to feel better.

Depression During Pregnancy Is Not Uncommon

Postpartum depression — depression after giving birth — has been well documented, with women like Brooke Shields and Drew Barrymore opening up to the media about their experiences. But antenatal depression — depression during pregnancy — still goes largely undiscussed, even though anywhere from 5 to 25 percent of pregnant women experience it.

There are a number of potential reasons for this. Women may be reluctant to reveal negative feelings at a time in their lives when society, family, and friends all expect them to be joyful. Women who are poor or who became pregnant unintentionally may regard symptoms of depression as a realistic response to their situation. Plus, some of the signs of depression — fatigue, changes in eating habits, sleep disturbances —are similar to the changes that many women experience as a typical part of pregnancy, making it harder to spot depression.

Therapists and physicians generally attempt to treat antenatal depression with non-medication methods first, as there is evidence that antidepressants may pose a risk to fetuses. For women with severe antenatal depression, however, antidepressants may be essential. Women need to educate themselves and work with their physicians to balance the risks and the benefits to both themselves and their infants.

SAD: When Depression Comes With the Seasons

A type of mild to severe depression that typically sets in as the hours of daylight wane in the fall, seasonal affective disorder (SAD) afflicts as many as six percents of Americans. Women are particularly at risk, experiencing SAD four times more often than men, as are people who have a relative with depression. People who live far from the equator tend to experience SAD in greater number 9 percent of Alaskans versus 1 percent of Floridians, according to the National Institute of Mental Health (NIMH).

The causes of SAD are unclear, says NIMH, but research suggests it may be due to seasonal fluctuations in levels of serotonin, a brain chemical that helps regulate mood, or to an overproduction of melatonin, the hormone that regulates sleep. Scientists also posit that people with SAD may produce too little vitamin D, which impacts serotonin activity.

For many people with SAD, simply waiting for spring to arrive is not an option. Light therapy, which generally involves sitting in front of a light box first thing in the morning, which can help, so can cognitive behavior therapy, a type of psychotherapy. Physicians also prescribe antidepressants, usually an SSRI (selective serotonin reuptake inhibitor), a category of drug that includes Prozac and Zoloft, or Wellbutrin (bupropion). Combining a number of different approaches under the oversight of a physician may be your smartest move.

Depression and Suicide Risk

A recent report from the Centers for Disease Control and Prevention (CDC) showed an increase in suicide among people not previously diagnosed with a mental disorder but there is a link between mental illness and suicide. Depression and other mental health conditions such as bipolar disorder, anxiety disorders, and schizophrenia are associated with an elevated risk for suicidal behavior. Among the symptoms associated with major depression are, recurrent thoughts of death and suicidal ideation with or without specific plans for committing suicide.

ADHD – Attention Deficit Hyperactivity Disorder

Attention Deficit Hyperactivity Disorder (ADHD) is a neurobiological condition that causes impulsivity, hyperactivity and inattention. This disorder can result in a number of behaviors that can hurt academic performance, including daydreaming in class, refusing to listen to others, fidgeting, constant talking and getting bored easily. Also, these students may make careless mistakes because of their impulsive nature or have trouble remembering when assignments are due. Compared to students without ADHD, students who live with the disorder are more likely to receive failing grades and lower grade point averages.

ADHD is frequently associated with other mental health issues, which can further contribute to challenges in school. Some students with ADHD also suffer from depression, anxiety or bipolar disorder.

What Is ADHD?

Attention deficit hyperactivity disorder (ADHD) is a chronic condition characterized by impulsive behaviour, inattention, and hyperactivity.

It's usually diagnosed in childhood, but symptoms of ADHD can continue through adolescence and adulthood, so it may also be diagnosed for the first time in adults. With proper treatment, children and adults with ADHD can live successful, highly productive lives.

What is the Difference Between ADHD and ADD?

Attention deficit disorder (ADD) is an older term for what's now known as ADHD. While some people still use the terms ADD and ADHD interchangeably, and may call the condition ADD if a child only has trouble focusing but isn't hyperactive, ADHD is officially recognized as the correct diagnosis of the condition by the current version of the American Psychiatric Association's Diagnostic and Statistical Manual of Mental Disorders (DSM).

The condition was commonly referred to as ADD until 1987 when "hyperactivity " was added to the name in the third edition of the DSM. When the revised, fourth edition of the DSM was published in 1994, ADHD was divided into specific subtypes, taking into account the fact that an individual could be diagnosed with ADHD without having symptoms of hyperactivity.

Types and Symptoms of ADHD

There are three forms — or "presentations" — of ADHD, as referred to in the DSM-5. The three are;

Predominantly Hyperactive-Impulsive

People with this type of ADHD mostly struggle with hyperactivity and impulsiveness, although they may also have some symptoms of inattentiveness.

Hyperactivity includes constant movement and excessive fidgeting and talking. In adults, this may take the form of exaggerated restlessness and an activity level that other people find tiring.

Impulsivity involves making important decisions and taking action without thinking through the consequences, especially when those actions might be harmful or detrimental and the effects long-lasting.

Impulsivity is also marked by a desire for instant gratification. In social situations, an impulsive person might interrupt others to an extreme degree, and be quick to grow impatient, frustrated, or angry.

Predominantly Inattentive

People in this category mainly have symptoms of inattentiveness, although they may still have some problems with hyperactivity and impulsiveness.

This form used to be (and sometimes still is) called ADD.

Inattentiveness is characterized by struggling to stay focused, being easily distracted from the task at hand, and a lack of persistence or organization. This can result in professional and personal difficulties — a lack of attention to detail and missing important deadlines, meetings, and social functions.

Combined Hyperactive-Impulsive and Inattentive

People in this group have symptoms of hyperactivity, impulsiveness, and inattentiveness. Most children have this combined type, but the most common symptom of ADHD in preschool-age children is hyperactivity.

Children who are hyperactive may talk excessively, squirm and fidget, and have trouble sitting still. In childhood, impulsivity can take the form of; impatience, disruptiveness, and difficulty waiting for a turn. Inattention can include; daydreaming, difficulty following instructions, forgetfulness in daily activities, and trouble focusing.

In adults, ADHD symptoms may take the form of; impulsiveness, frequent interrupting, restlessness, inability to concentrate, a lack of organization and follow-through, difficulty meeting deadlines, frequent mood swings, and struggling to cope with stress.

How Is ADHD Diagnosed?

Though many people lose focus, get distracted, and act impulsively on occasion, these behaviors are more severe and more frequent for people with ADHD. Without proper identification and treatment, these behaviors negatively affect their quality of life, whether it's at work, school, or home.

There isn't a standardised test that fits all type of ADHD test to diagnose the disorder. A thorough evaluation by a professional — such as a psychologist, psychiatrist, pediatrician, or clinical social worker — is necessary for a proper diagnosis, which rules out other conditions and considers possible co-existing conditions.

The process involves several steps and your healthcare provider may perform a full medical exam and get a detailed medical history, as well as conduct interviews with family members to gather a personal history.

The DSM now requires that ADHD diagnoses include the severity of the condition, from mild to moderate to severe.

How ADHD Affects Children

ADHD affects more than 10 percent of school-aged children. According to the Centers for Disease Control and Prevention, 14.2 percent of boys and 6.4 percent of girls have been diagnosed with ADHD.

ADHD is more frequently diagnosed in boys, but research suggests that it may be under-identified and under-diagnosed in girls.

A study published in the journal BMC Psychiatry in November 2013, notes that girls more commonly present behaviour the coincides with the inattentive subtype of ADHD and that their behavior may sometimes be characterized as less outwardly disruptive. Many women don't receive a proper diagnosis until they are adults.

Kids with the disorder typically have symptoms that cause

problems at home, at school, or in social situations. Parents and teachers often mistake signs of ADHD for emotional or behavioral problems.

How ADHD Affects Adults

ADHD affects more than 4 percent of adults in the United States, according to the National Institute of Mental Health. But that statistic doesn't include adults who may have ADHD but haven't been diagnosed.

More than 75 percent of children with ADHD continue to experience significant symptoms in adulthood, according to the organization Children and Adults With Attention-Deficit/Hyperactivity Disorder (CHADD).

Adults with ADHD may sometimes struggle with relationships, work performance, and self-esteem. Many adults with ADHD don't even know they have it; they may only know that everyday tasks are challenging for them, but they may not question why.

Symptoms can change over time. Some people notice that their symptoms improve as they age, while others continue to struggle.

According to Russell Barkley, Ph.D., a clinical professor of psychiatry at the Virginia Treatment Center for Children and the Virginia Commonwealth University Medical Center in Richmond, Virginia, ADHD symptoms arise in a set of mental abilities called the executive functions.

The executive functions encompass a range of processes in the brain, mostly in the frontal areas, that control and manage other brain activities that allow us to get work done — whether its creative or more routine; to set and achieve goals, and to take into consideration the potential consequences of our actions and regulate our behaviour.

Dr. Barkley, the author of Attention Deficit Hyperactivity Disorders: A Handbook for Diagnosis and Treatment (Guilford Press, 2014) breaks this down into several areas, including self-awareness, inhibition or self-restraint, working memory (meaning actively keeping in mind what you are supposed to be doing in order to achieve a goal or complete a task), time management, emotional self-control, self-motivation, and planning or problem-solving.

Causes and Risk Factors for ADHD

Experts aren't sure what causes ADHD. Research suggests that the disorder has a strong neurobiological basis and that heredity is a major factor.

Neuroimaging studies using MRIs to look at brain structure have found a consistent set of neural circuits to be associated with ADHD. These circuits are related to sustained attention, control of inhibitions, motivation, and regulation of emotions.

But it's unclear whether ADHD behaviours result from abnormal neural connections or whether there is a neural adaptation because of symptoms.

Imaging studies have shown that certain areas of the brain are smaller in children with ADHD compared with children who don't have ADHD. Two meta-analyses found that these differences in brain volume are no longer detectable in adulthood, suggesting that ADHD symptoms may be due, in part, to delays in development or maturation.

Several factors may increase a child's likelihood of developing ADHD:

Genetics appear to play the largest role. ADHD has been shown to run in families, and studies have estimated that heritability may range from 60 to 90 percent.

Although the specific genes at play have not yet been identified, scientists believe multiple genes may be involved, because it's such a complex condition. These genes may have to do with the processes of certain neurotransmitters, such as dopamine, which plays a role in the brain's reward systems and in regulating impulsivity and movement.

Environmental exposure to toxins and chemicals, especially to lead, may be a contributing factor. Studies have indicated a relationship between ADHD and levels of lead in the bloodstream. One 2010 study, published in the Journal of Child Psychology and Psychiatry, found that lead exposure was associated with the impulsivity-hyperactivity combined type of ADHD but not the inattentive type.

Alcohol or tobacco use during pregnancy has been associated with with ADHD symptoms in children in some studies. But more recent research has questioned whether the use of these substances directly causes ADHD.

A study published in April 2016 in the Journal of Child Psychology and Psychiatry found no support for a causal association between smoking during pregnancy and ADHD. Similarly, a study published in October 2017 in the International Journal of Epidemiology found that maternal alcohol use during pregnancy was weakly, though perhaps causally, associated with reported ADHD symptoms but not with clinical diagnoses of ADHD.

Still, pregnant women should refrain from alcohol consumption and smoking because of other well-established risks.

Traumatic brain injury (TBI) in early childhood has been linked to the development of psychiatric disorders. Among those disorders, ADHD is the most common, with a prevalence of about 20 percent, notes a study published in March 2018 in JAMA Pediatrics. (17)

TBI is not uncommon — more than 1 million children and young adults seek emergency treatment for it each year.

Premature birth or low birth weight may increase the risk of ADHD. Some research has suggested a correlation along a gradient — that the lower the birth weight or, the higher the preterm level, the greater the risk of ADHD. A meta-analysis and review of 34 studies, published in January 2018 in Pediatrics confirmed this, showing an even stronger association with the development of ADHD when birth weight was extremely low or the birth was extremely preterm (which the World Health Organization defines as before 28 weeks. (18)

Diet and behavioral factors such as consuming too much sugar or food additives or excessive screen time (television, smartphones, tablets, and computers) have been associated with ADHD. While these factors may affect or exacerbate symptoms, research doesn't support claims that they cause ADHD.

ADHD Complications and Comorbidities

Untreated ADHD can lead to several emotional and physical complications, including:

- Poor self-esteem
- Accidents and injuries
- Substance abuse
- Delinquent or risky behaviour
- Trouble interacting with peers; relationship

difficulties
- Excess weight and eating disorders
- Sleeping problems

More than two-thirds of people with ADHD have at least one other coexisting condition, whose symptoms can sometimes be hard to distinguish from those of ADHD.

Children with ADHD may be more likely to have other conditions, such as:

- Anxiety
- Learning disabilities
- Depression
- Bipolar disorder, a condition characterized by periods of depression and manic behaviour
- Oppositional defiant disorder (ODD), a condition characterized by a pattern of hostile behavior toward authority figures
- Conduct disorder, a condition characterized by behaviours such as lying, stealing, fighting, or bullying
- Tourette's syndrome, a neurological disorder

characterized by nervous tics and repetitive mannerisms
- Sleep disorders
- Bed-wetting

Treatment for ADHD

There's no cure for ADHD, but the right treatment approach can help control many symptoms. This usually involves taking medication, learning certain behavioral strategies, and implementing lifestyle changes to help with focus and organization.

For children under six with ADHD, the American Academy of Pediatrics (AAP) recommends behavioral therapy as the first line of treatment, before medication.

Medication is recommended for children six years of age and older. Medications used for treating ADHD include stimulants, nonstimulants, and sometimes antidepressants.

People with ADHD may also benefit from counselling — especially behavioral therapy — to improve behaviors and social skills. Parents and other family members may participate in counseling to help develop strategies for dealing with problematic situations.

Certain lifestyle changes and accommodations can create a better environment for people with ADHD. These include routines and schedules, reorganization of your home or workspace, physical reminders of tasks at hand, and removal of distractions.

Proper, comprehensive treatment can help control ADHD symptoms and lead to an improved quality of life.

PTSD- Post-Traumatic Stress Disorder

Post-Traumatic Stress Disorder (PTSD) can occur when someone experiences a traumatic stressor in their life. While people often think of PTSD as something that only affects veterans coping with their experiences on the battlefield, the condition can be caused by some traumatic experiences — such as serious accidents, domestic abuse, assaults or non-violent crime. Also, PTSD can also be caused by witnessing a traumatic event.

PTSD can have serious effects on the brain that impair memory and make it difficult for students to do well in school. Also, these students may also experience panic attacks and a lack of motivation or concentration, as well as disordered sleeping and eating patterns. All of these symptoms make it difficult for students to pay attention in class and keep up with their assignments, potentially leading to poor grades.

Post-Traumatic Stress Disorder

PTSD is a disorder that develops in some people who have experienced a shocking, scary, or dangerous event.

It is natural to feel afraid during and after a traumatic situation. Fear triggers many split-second changes in the body to help defend against danger or to avoid it. This "fight-or-flight" response is a typical reaction meant to protect a person from harm. Nearly everyone will experience a range of reactions after trauma, yet most people recover from initial symptoms naturally. Those who continue to experience problems may be diagnosed with PTSD. People who have PTSD may feel stressed or frightened even when they are not in danger.

Signs and Symptoms

Not every traumatized person develops ongoing (chronic) or even short-term (acute) PTSD. Not everyone with PTSD has been through a dangerous event. Some experiences, like the sudden, unexpected death of a loved one, can also cause PTSD. Symptoms usually begin early, within three months of the traumatic incident, but sometimes they begin years afterward. Symptoms must last more than a month and be severe enough to interfere with relationships or work to be considered PTSD. The course of the illness varies. Some people recover within six months, while others have symptoms that last much longer. In some people, the condition becomes chronic.

A doctor who has experience helping people with mental illnesses, such as a psychiatrist or psychologist, can diagnose PTSD.

To be diagnosed with PTSD, an adult must have all of the following for at least one month:

- At least one re-experiencing symptom
- At least one avoidance symptom
- At least two arousal and reactivity symptoms
- At least two cognition and mood symptoms

Re-experiencing symptoms include:

- Flashbacks—reliving the trauma over and over, including physical symptoms like a racing heart or sweating
- Bad dreams
- Frightening thoughts

Re-experiencing symptoms may cause problems in a person's everyday routine. The symptoms can start from the person's thoughts and feelings. Words, objects, or situations that are reminders of the event can also trigger re-experiencing symptoms.

Avoidance symptoms include:

- Staying away from places, events, or objects that are reminders of the traumatic experience
- Avoiding thoughts or feelings related to the traumatic event

Things that remind a person of the traumatic event can trigger avoidance symptoms. These symptoms may cause a person to change his or her personal routine. For example, after a bad car accident, a person who usually drives may avoid driving or ride in a car.

Arousal and reactivity symptoms include:

- Being easily startled
- Feeling tense or "on edge"
- Having difficulty sleeping
- Having angry outbursts

Arousal symptoms are usually constant, instead of being triggered by things that remind one of the traumatic events. These symptoms can make the person feel stressed and angry. They may make it hard to do daily tasks, such as sleeping, eating, or concentrating.

Cognition and mood symptoms include:

- Trouble remembering the key features of the traumatic event
- Negative thoughts about oneself or the world
- Distorted feelings like guilt or blame
- Loss of interest in enjoyable activities

Cognition and mood symptoms can begin or worsen after the traumatic event but are not due to injury or substance use. These symptoms can make the person feel alienated or detached from friends or family members.

It is natural to have some of these symptoms after a dangerous event. Sometimes people have very serious symptoms that go away after a few weeks. This is called acute stress disorder, or ASD. When the symptoms last more than a month, seriously affect one's ability to function, and are not due to substance use, medical illness, or anything except the event itself, they might be PTSD. Some people with PTSD don't show any symptoms for weeks or months. PTSD is often accompanied by depression, substance abuse, or one or more of the other anxiety disorders.

Do children react differently than adults?

Children and teens can have extreme reactions to trauma, but their symptoms may not be the same as adults. In very young children (less than six years of age), these symptoms can include:

- Wetting the bed after having learned to use the toilet
- Forgetting how to or being unable to talk
- Acting out the scary event during playtime
- Being unusually clingy with a parent or other adult

Older children and teens are more likely to show symptoms similar to those seen in adults. They may also develop disruptive, disrespectful, or destructive behaviours. Older children and teens may feel guilty for not preventing injury or deaths. They may also have thoughts of revenge. For additional information, visit the Learn More section below. The National Institute of Mental Health (NIMH) offers free print materials in English and Spanish. These can be read online, downloaded, or delivered to you in the mail.

Risk Factors

Anyone can develop PTSD at any age. This includes war veterans, children, and people who have been through a physical or sexual assault, abuse, accident, disaster, or many other serious events. According to the National Center for PTSD, about 7 or 8 out of every 100 people will experience PTSD at some point in their lives. Women are more likely to develop PTSD than men, and genes may make some people more likely to develop PTSD than others.

Not everyone with PTSD has been through a dangerous event. Some people develop PTSD after a friend or family member experiences danger or harm. The sudden, unexpected death of a loved one can also lead to PTSD.

Why do some people develop PTSD and other people do not?

It is important to remember that not everyone who lives through a dangerous event develops PTSD. In fact, most people will not develop the disorder.

Many factors play a part in whether a person will develop PTSD. Some examples are listed below. Risk factors make a person more likely to develop PTSD. Other factors, called resilience factors, can help reduce the risk of the disorder.

Risk Factors and Resilience Factors for PTSD

Some factors that increase the risk for PTSD include:

- Living through dangerous events and traumas
- Getting hurt
- Seeing another person hurt, or seeing a dead body
- Childhood trauma
- Feeling horror, helplessness, or extreme fear
- Having little or no social support after the event
- Dealing with extra stress after the event, such as loss of a loved one, pain and injury, or loss of a job or home

- Having a history of mental illness or substance abuse
- Some resilience factors that may reduce the risk of PTSD include:
- Seeking out support from other people, such as friends and family
- Finding a support group after a traumatic event
- Learning to feel good about one's actions in the face of danger
- Having, a positive coping strategy, or a way of getting through the bad event and learning from it
- Being able to act and respond effectively despite feeling fear

Researchers are studying the importance of these and other risk and resilience factors, including genetics and neurobiology. With more research, someday it may be possible to predict who is likely to develop PTSD and to prevent it.

Treatments and Therapies

The main treatments for people with PTSD are medications, psychotherapy ("talk" therapy), or both. Everyone is different, and PTSD affects people differently so a treatment that works for one person may not work for another. It is important for anyone with PTSD to be treated by a mental health provider who is experienced with PTSD. Some people with PTSD need to try different treatments to find what works for their symptoms.

If someone with PTSD is going through an ongoing trauma, such as being in an abusive relationship, both of the problems need to be addressed. Other ongoing problems can include panic disorder, depression, substance abuse, and feeling suicidal.

Medications

The most studied medications for treating PTSD include antidepressants, which may help control PTSD symptoms such as sadness, worry, anger, and feeling numb inside. Antidepressants and other medications may be prescribed along with psychotherapy. Other medications may be helpful for specific PTSD symptoms. For example, although it is not currently FDA approved, research has shown that Prazosin may be helpful with sleep problems, particularly nightmares, commonly experienced by people with PTSD.

Doctors and patients can work together to find the best medication or medication combination, as well as the right dose.

Psychotherapy

Psychotherapy (sometimes called "talk therapy") involves talking with a mental health professional to treat mental illness. Psychotherapy can occur one-on-one or in a group. Talk therapy treatment for PTSD usually lasts 6 to 12 weeks, but it can last longer. Research shows that support from family and friends can be an important part of recovery.

Many types of psychotherapy can help people with PTSD. Some types target the symptoms of PTSD directly. Other therapies focus on social, family, or job-related problems.

The doctor or therapist may combine different therapies depending on each person's needs.

Effective psychotherapies tend to emphasize a few key components, including education about symptoms, teaching skills to help identify the triggers of symptoms, and skills to manage the symptoms. One helpful form of therapy is called cognitive behavioural therapy, or CBT. CBT can include:

- Exposure therapy. This helps people face and control their fear. It gradually exposes them to the trauma they experienced in a safe way. It uses imagining, writing, or visiting the place where the event happened. The therapist uses these tools to help people with PTSD cope with their feelings.
- Cognitive restructuring. This helps people make sense of the bad memories. Sometimes people remember the event differently than how it happened. They may feel guilt or shame about something that is, not their fault. The therapist helps people with PTSD look at what happened in a realistic way.

There are other types of treatment that can help as well. People with PTSD should talk about all treatment options with a therapist. Treatment should equip individuals with the skills to manage their symptoms and help them participate in activities that they enjoyed before developing PTSD.

How Talk Therapies Help People Overcome PTSD

Talk therapies teach people helpful ways to react to the frightening events that trigger their PTSD symptoms. Based on this general goal, different types of therapy may:

- Teach about trauma and its effects
- Use relaxation and anger-control skills
- Provide tips for better sleep, diet, and exercise habits
- Help people identify and deal with guilt, shame, and other feelings about the event
- Focus on changing how people react to their PTSD symptoms. For example, therapy helps people face reminders of the trauma.

Beyond Treatment: How can I help myself?

It may be very hard to take that first step to help yourself. It is important to realize that although it may take some time, with treatment, you can get better. If you are unsure where to go for help, ask your family doctor. You can also check NIMH's Help for Mental Illnesses page or search online for "mental health providers", "social services", "hotlines", or "physicians" for phone numbers and addresses. An emergency room doctor can also provide temporary help and can tell you where and how to get further help.

To help yourself while in treatment:

- Talk with your doctor about treatment options
- Engage in mild physical activity or exercise to help reduce stress
- Set realistic goals for yourself
- Break up large tasks into small ones, set some priorities, and do what you can as you can
- Try to spend time with other people, and confide in a trusted friend or relative. Tell others about things that may trigger symptoms

- Expect your symptoms to improve gradually, not immediately
- Identify and seek out comforting situations, places, and people

Caring for yourself and others are especially important when large numbers of people are exposed to traumatic events (such as natural disasters, accidents, and violent acts). For, more information, see the Learn More section, below.

11: Does Getting Good Sleep Affect Our Ability to Stay Healthy?

Modern researchers tell us that few people sleep well anymore. However, sleep is all important in having a well-rounded successful and healthy life.

Good sleep means one's body undergoes all four sleep cycles to be considered complete--alpha, beta, delta, and theta. Furthermore, doctors advise us to get at least eight hours of this good sleep per night. For various reasons, many of us get much less rest than that. (Keep in mind that sleep is not merely a state of not being awake.)

So, while in grad school, you might just feel everything is going wrong and you are not stable mentally.

Check to see if you have been having a good sleep.

A natural cycle of rest and wakefulness dictates all sorts of biological functions,

Sleep loss is associated with the following:

- Heart disease
- Diabetes

- Cancer
- Obesity
- Depression
- Infections
- Accidents

Wikipedia defines sleep as "the state of natural rest... a protective mechanism... and also necessary for health and survival". Upon close inspection, sleep not only drops our conscious mind into a deep state of relaxation and rest, but scores of biochemical mechanisms are busily, yet quietly functioning inside. A portion of the body is not really at rest, even during the deepest of sleep.

What Happens During Sleep?

1. Damage to cells, tissues, and organs is repaired. Cells do not live forever, and those cells which cannot be saved are subject to apoptosis or cell death. The body systematically rids you of those cells every day and prepares the body to excrete them. This is excellent and necessary internal housekeeping. The body rids itself of unwanted, non-

functioning and abnormal cells while it aggressively makes new, healthy ones. Sleep is prime time for your body to concentrate on these important changes.

2. Substances such as bio-chemicals, blood products, and bone marrow are manufactured while you sleep. As the body slows down during rest, it replenishes these vital, life-sustaining components. Example: When you catch an infectious agent, and blood components are needed for the Immune System to combat the invader, this system of renewal generates necessary immune fighting cells for the body. This alleviates your system of trying to fight off the infection from a weakened, sub-standard state. Your Immune System and every system of the body must be strong. They get this necessary support if your body gets the daily rest that it needs!

3. The unconscious mind processes the day's events. This is an important function if you want to have good mental health and be able to handle stress well. Lack of good quality sleep is an attributing factor to depression and

some forms of mental illness. One finds serious sleep disorders in untreated people. And let's not forget about the importance of dreaming; it is the mechanism which allows the unconscious mind to play. Medicine considers this is an important brain function and non-dreamers are cheated of this delightful luxury!

4. As you rest, the body renews its energy stores for the next day. We all need to regenerate new energy reserves thus enabling us to tackle each day. However, people living with compromised health, unresolved traumas, and extreme tension or those living in unsafe environments rarely wake up feeling rested. Some only nap and never really sleep at all (especially chronically ill people). People with this problem build larger and larger sleep deficits; they never get caught up. If a normal sleep pattern ultimately cannot be restored, a person's health will continue to decline. When sleep can be normalized, and this one issue is a valuable aid in total recovery from illness.

Okay. Let's agree that sleep is important from a normal physical and disease prevention standpoint, but does an altered sleep mechanism impact other types of health issues? What about people who seem to need extraordinary amounts of sleep?

Sleep for Healing

People who suffer from life-altering illness or who are recovering from trauma instinctively know that they need sleep - sometimes, lots of it. Their bodies require extraordinary amounts of rest to facilitate the healing process. If your body is fighting infections, if you have compromised organ systems or if you're fighting chronic pain, this is especially true.

Take this bit of advice into your being. Determine today how critical it is to sleep well and live a healthy lifestyle. You want to be free of disease and chronic health problems!

12: Boost Your Mental Health With The Brain Games!

With the growing age, the brain also starts fading. By the time, you turn 30 years of age, your brain starts aging. Don't panic! There is a solution to this problem - Brain games for students. It is a difficult situation when too much of studying and stress starts affecting your brain, and you get infested with some or the other memory-related disease. One of the major mental diseases which have affected students in the distant past is dementia or Alzheimer's. A very dangerous mental disorder which is incurable! But definitely, the effect can be reduced with some measures like doing regular brain exercises. There are numerous brain games designed, especially for the adults. Using these brain teasers in your daily routine tasks, you can actually reduce a lot of mental burdens and can put your brain to test.

Fighting any disease with medical aid is the ultimate solution, but if you have a better and a more convenient solution then why not opt for it. Now, this is when playing those brain games for adults become essential. Fix up time and follow that every day, if not possible every day then at least every alternate day. If you give reasons that you don't have time to do that, then I must say that it is an excuse. If you are willing to do something, you can actually do that. These brain games not only help the adults to a great extent in their day-to-day activities but rather improve their ability to handle work at home and office with equal efficiency. If you are facing some memory related issues like short memory loss, forgetting the recently observed facts and data or the inability to acquire new memories, etc. you need help. Start using these brain games for adults. They are truly magical; it is being seen that people who are regular with their memory refining regime are healthier and more active.

With adults, the kids also have their concerns, which if tackled on time will show minimal bad effects. If your kid is not very active and sharp, give them the gift of these educational school games. These games are specially designed for the kids; this helps in improving their general knowledge, their mathematical and logical skills and so much more. In schools also, teachers are very particular about these educational games as this helps in the overall personality enrichment. Without wasting any time, purchase these educational school games for your kids and help them grow as smarter and sharper individuals.

PART THREE: TIME MANAGEMENT

13: Learning Time Management Skills

Learning, time management skills, are like any other skill in that it takes time to develop them and you must make regular use of them to keep them sharp. Depending on your job or life people often focus on different aspects of time management, but here we will focus on learning time management skills that most people will find useful.

1. The top skill is to learn to focus on what is most meaningful for you today. Most people get caught up in trying to accomplish trivial tasks so they can feel good about crossing them off the to-do list. What you need to do is focus on what one or two tasks are most important for you to do that day and get them done first. Time management often comes down to a mental state of whether or not you feel like you are in control of your time.

2. The second skill to learn is long-term time management. Where do you want to be six months from now? By knowing that answer, it should dictate what you need to accomplish today. Set your long-term goals and then break them down into weekly or daily tasks, so you are gradually

building towards them.

3. The third and some might argue the most important skill is the daily review. At the end of the day examine what you accomplished that day. Ask yourself about what parts of the day you managed efficiently and what parts you did not. By just doing this one time management skill daily you can rapidly accomplish any goal. As the famous quote says 'an unexamined life is not worth living.'

4. The fourth major time management skill to learn is having a commitment to continued learning. As you advance in your career and life the time management skills that got you where you are will likely not get you to where you want to go. So by learning new skills on a regular basis, you can continue advancing in your management of time.

By focusing on learning time management skills like the ones we talked about above you too can master time management. Your focus every day should be continual and gradual improvement in your time management skills. Once you do this long enough, it should become a habit that can lead you to even greater success in life.

14: Time Management Skills - Why They Are Important

Have you ever wished there were more than 24 hours in a day? Have you ever wished you could be in two places at the same time? Have you ever felt so stressed that you want to scream? Maybe you have actually screamed!

Does it seem like you always have done too many things at once and not enough time to do them? It seems like no matter how hard you work, you still do not get everything done.

So what is it? Why is it that you feel so stressed? You picked up all the skills you needed to excel in your chosen profession. You do a great job, yet you feel rushed. You feel like there is so much to do.

This is where time management skills play such an important role. If you learn this skill, then you will be able to feel a lot less stressed. You will find that you will be a lot more productive and accomplish a lot more in less time.

In school, you are taught math, science and English. But you are not taught to manage your time. Even though it is one of the most important skills in life, it is the one that you are not taught.

Some people eventually realize that they need to learn this skill. They then go out and educate themselves.

There are many people though that never realize what is stopping them from leading a stress-free life. They continue to have too much to do and continue to feel like a hamster in a wheel.

If you have ever met someone who you think is superman or superwoman, just ask them how they do it. To you, it seems as if they have a magic touch. They get everything done and are still calm and happy.

Yes, they do have a magic touch. And that magic touch is time management skills. Ask them, and they will tell you the same thing. If you want to have a stress-free, calm life you have to learn that important magic touch - time management skills.

How to Learn Time Management Skills

Time Management is a challenging task for most of the

people. It can be defined as the best possible way to utilize available time. It enables you to perform and accomplish tasks at the right time. Time management plays a significant role in your professional and personal life. It includes six phases, which are listed below:

- Effective planning
- Setting short and long-term goals
- Setting deadlines
- Assigning responsibilities
- Prioritizing activities as per the importance
- Spending time on the right activities as per their importance

There are various potential benefits of time management that encourage people to think about it and managing their time accordingly. One needs to be motivated to make the necessary changes to improve the quality of his/her life. This innovative skill can be learned easily. Some of the key advantages of time management skills are as follow:

Reduce stress

In several situations, poor work habits lead to stress. For instance, eating on the run or while watching TV, leaving tasks or things for the last minute, working for hours without taking a break, etc. When you start managing your time by scheduling and prioritizing your tasks, you instantly feel less stressed and calmer. The on-time accomplishment of assignments or tasks reduces your stress level.

Improve productivity

The unorganized schedule often causes confusion, lots of incomplete work and less time. It is difficult to meet your professional and personal goals when you fail to manage your daily schedule. It is important to know what is needed to be done and when it should become completed in order to achieve your personal goals. Prepare a to-do-list and schedule your time accordingly.

Gaining control

When you begin switching from one task to another without any delay because of constantly changing priorities, urgent tasks and crises, you immediately feel very helpless. Some people may try to get into your schedule until you don't have enough space for your own. The effective time management provides you perfect control over your tasks like what you are doing and when you suppose to finish it.

Build confidence

Confidence is the foundation and most important aspect of life. Managing things according to your to-do-list and planned schedule build your confidence by making you realize you achieve what you aspired. When you gain control over your personal and professional life, you feel more confident.

Sense of Achievement

When you know, you can accomplish all tasks without the

hassle and stress that needed to be done. The result is more worthy and something you can proud of.

Peace of mind

With proper scheduling, you will realize that you have enough time to perform various other leisure activities as well. You will feel more relaxed and calm. It avoids you from the constant worries like how to get it done, will it be finished on time, etc. When you are not in a hurry and overworked, you feel a sense of peace, called peace of mind.

Some Reasons Why You May Exhibit Poor Time Management Skills

There Are Several Reasons Why

Some people may have poor home time management skills and, from my experience, these are the most common. See if you see yourself in one of these categories but know, even if you do, there's still hope.

1 - You never learned home time management skills

It's really hard to learn home time management skills when you're so busy putting out fire after fire. By the time you've taken off your Fire Chief's helmet, you're too exhausted to think about where that next hotspot will flare up. So, inevitably, you start out the next morning with... I can already guess... a new fire to put out. It's a vicious cycle but one which, fortunately, can be broken.

How? Start paying attention to the future more. Begin on Monday night to think about Tuesday. What do you have to do? What are you going to fix for dinner? Do the kids have any kind of practice? Think, plan, and think some more. The more you practice this, the better you'll get.

I've found that, for me, weekly planning is the best because it allows me to plan yet it's not so in advance that it's unstable.

2 - You never had to manage your time wisely

I know it's hard to believe, but some people are so spoilt that they have no concept of home time management.

They may not have to get up and go to a job or school, or they may just be lazy. I knew one woman who had been a housewife for many years... let me rephrase that... she didn't work outside of the home or inside it either. When her husband left her, she had absolutely no concept of time management. Now that was work to get her straightened out! Severe laziness can be overcome.

How? Find out what will motivate you. Create a list of goals. When we have goals we're working towards, then we're motivated to find the time to work on them. Having to find time for something usually means learning and then utilizing home time management skills.

3 - Learning home time management skills was too much work

You just never wanted to expend the energy to learn and then practice new skills. It always seemed like too much time to make those monthly menus or create that family calendar. Maybe now your life has changed, and you need those long put off skills. You can get them at last.

How? Take the time to concentrate on one aspect at a time. Since you spend a lot of time in the kitchen, learn how to create weekly menus first off then you can graduate to something else.

Time Management Skills - Unlocking Your Potential

First and foremost are superior time management skills. Time management allows you to achieve what you set out to do every day. Superior time management skills allow time for bumps in the road that may alter your daily course, without falling off track completely. The key to handling the work load you are given is evaluating what is currently on your plate and weighing it against the new task as hand. Depending on the outcome, you may need to learn how to say "no" every once in a while, or at least "not right now".

The second tool in your business skill arsenal is organization. This goes hand-in-hand with time management but presents with it a new set of obstacles. You see, in order to be organized, you have to manage your time wisely. You must be able to fit everything you say you are going to do into the period given for turn around. That said, you can't necessarily be rigid in the organization style you utilize. More often than not, things are going to crop up throughout a day which can cause you to detour from your original plan of attack. Roll with the punches, and allow for these obstacles to be overcome by marrying these two top business skills together. A way to tackle them is by planning for these time traps by allowing some unscheduled or free time at different intervals during the course of your day. In this way, you allow yourself the needed window in case something should come up to fill it.

These are just two of the many top business skills seen in today's workforce leaders. The key to discovering the right ones for your needs is to analyze where you desire to be and who in that field you look up to. Once identified, the world is your oyster. You simply need to step forth and show the world the treasure which you alone possess.

Time Management Skills: The Benefits

People with good time management skills are more likely to be successful in their lives. There are many benefits to having good time management skills. In general, you are more effective in getting your work done. You can stop being reactive in your life and start working productively towards your goals. When you have good time management skills, you aren't wasting time, and you are able to manage your resources better. Tasks get done faster, and then you have more time to relax, and enjoy life, or move onto the next task.

If you own your own business "time wasted equals money lost". If you are able to manage your time better, you can make massive improvements in how your business is run. It will be more effective, and that means more profit! You can also have more time to be with your family. You can be the work at home mom and benefit from your superior time management skills.

While these are all good benefits, time manage can bring an even greater one into your life: Happiness. Your lifestyle is overall less stressful and more profitable. Your lifestyle and business can both improve from having good time management skills.

Once you have effective time management skills, you will be able to see where you are wasting your time in everyday life. When you see where your time is being wasted, you can improve it. Time management also teaches you about priorities. We can see which priorities are higher on the list than others. There are certain things in life that cannot be avoided; these things should rank lower on your list of priorities. These events you more than likely can put off for another day. It is important that you separate the events that need to be done from the events that you can do tomorrow.

Creating a list of priorities is essential in maintaining good time management. If you follow the proper schedules and routines, you should become effective with your time. The most important thing you have to do is stick with your plan. If you find that is too difficult to do, you might want to consider readjusting it, for it might be too unrealistic. If you keep good time management skills, your life, in general, will become more relaxed and less stressful. Overall, good time management skills are an essential quality in life.

Time Management Skills - Learn the Secret of Good Time Management Skills

How often do you hear people saying that they are struggling to meet their deadlines or do everything they want to do within the available time? I guess many of you will say this is a common problem of life and one that will always be with humanity forever. I would have believed this to be the case had I not been privileged to meet people who are experts in managing their time effectively to meet their personal and professional goals consistently. These rare time management experts are masters in employing strategies for minimizing time-wasting activities as part of their daily routines and moreover have a strong habit of focusing their energy and attention toward maximizing the use of their time doing important and urgent activities link directly to their personal and professional goals. Regardless of whether you are in business or in employment time management strategies will help you achieve the best use of your time. In this article, some of the strategies employed by time management experts will be uncovered.

Before progressing into the meaty aspect of this subject,

let me start by asking you two basic questions. What is your disposition towards "Time"? Do you see time as a resource to be valued just like money? Whatever your response to these questions, I am sure we will all agree on one thing, "Time" is non-discriminatory. Regardless of our geographical locations, creed, color or ethnicity, everyone has access to 24 hours dosages of "Time". So, how can you ensure you use your time wisely to achieve your personal or professional goals? The simple answer to this is "Learn the secret of good time management skills".

Time management is the art of managing one's time effectively doing things that are important and urgent. It is about prioritizing our activities such that we focus on the things that are important to us based on our judgment.

This implies that the first strategy to eliminate poor time management is to determine very clearly what is important to us regarding our personal and professional goals and then to take concrete steps to be involved in activities that will directly or indirectly contribute to the accomplishment of our all-important personal and professional goals. This sounds very simple in theory, but the truth is that in practice this can be very difficult to implement. This is because in practice most people do not consciously set themselves personal and professional goals for life and as a result, they tend to allow the rest of the world to shape the direction of their daily activities and goals.

The second strategy that can facilitate an effective use of "Time" is the use of effective planning systems to guide our daily activities. Time management experts are masters of planning their activities. They pre-plan what needs be done, by whom and when often well in advance of the events. As a result, they are able to work around distractions outside their planned activities. Let me quickly add a qualification here; do understand that time management does not advocate rigidity with plans that are clearly unworkable. The important point to bear in mind is that planning can help us prevent people dumping activities on us that are outside the sphere of our important personal and professional goals so long as we are able to compliment the planning skills with assertive skills. There is an old proverb which goes like this: "If you do not plan what you want to do someone else will plan what you should be doing". On the subject of assertive skills, this is critical if you are going to be able to manage your plans leading to your personal and professional goals. So let's just explore this concept further. Being assertive simply means understanding your rights and respecting the rights of others. Consequently, assertive people do not allow others to violate their rights and are able to say "NO" to unreasonable requests and demands on their time. It is precisely for this reason, and time management experts are able to decline requests over and beyond their personal capacity, whereas those lacking in this skills accept every request made on their time only to find themselves stressed and frustrated.

At Business Services Support Limited, we have developed an easy to read the booklet on the subject of Time Management For Busy Managers. We also run a training workshop on time management skills. If you would like to find out more about time management resources, articles and seminars on time management contact us today.

Improve Time Management Skill - Identify Your Greatest Obstacles

The desire to improve time management skills is coveted

by many if recent searches on the Internet are even a remotely accurate assessment of this desire. From the Internet and all the local public workshops and seminars, there appears that many are desirous of learning time management skills. So, if the desire is great and the supply is equally great, then why do so many people still have time management challenges?

First, time management is not about managing time since time is a constant. Second, today's society is experiencing more change in one year than their grandparents faced during their entire lifetimes. Finally, time management is truly about self-management or self-leadership skills.

If we begin to improve time management skills by looking at time management from a different perspective, we then can begin to realize positive behavioral changes. From these changes, we can see improved results.

Now that you understand that time management is not about time, but rather is about how we handle change through our self-leadership skills, we begin to identify those obstacles keeping us from improved results. So, what are your obstacles?

After speaking to and working with hundreds of individuals, I have come to realize that to improve time management skills requires that we must have a proven goal setting process and a written goals action plan. For without goals, why do we care if we are on time or not?

Another obstacle to effective time management skills is attitudes or those habits of thoughts. Do you wake up knowing exactly what you need to do first because the night before you plan your next day? Or do you wait to the last minute to see what you are doing in the next hour or two? Poor attitudes are demonstrated through poor behaviours.

Because self-leadership skills are weak such as decision making, prioritizing, communicating, etc., these deficiencies have a negative impact on the ability to improve time management skills When a plan is put in place to improve self-leadership skills, time management skills will also improve.

If you want to improve your time management skills, then look to:

- Committing your goals to write and putting them into

a goals action plan
- Determining what attitudes are obstacles standing in your way
- Developing self-leadership skills that will support your ability to handle change
- By identifying and removing these obstacles, you will improve time management skills and have a much more successful life.

The 4 Must-Have Time Management Skills

You may be wondering how some people can play so many different roles in life in so little time. Their secret in living such a life is not actually a secret; it is just simply a matter of obtaining great time management skills. Fortunately, you do not have to be living so many roles just to be able to able to have these excellent skills; you just have to practice some of the things that will be discussed here.

Unlike managing your work desk, practicing time management skills takes some patience, perseverance, and self-control because it is not just a matter of having some physical changes; it is more of a mental transformation - a change in one's behavior.

One of the things that you must practice if you are to manage your time efficiently is to learn how to say no. Once you have already planned your day ahead, hold on to it as tight and as reasonably as you can. Take this example: You are planning to finish your weekend report today but your friends drop by with their car and they are inviting you to a party right on the spot. When this happens, do not hesitate to say no - no matter how much they tease you about being workaholic or lame; just stick to your plans, and by doing so, you save more time for more productive things, and you also earn your friends' respect both at the same time.

If you are already at the exact time where you are planning to start something, then start, regardless whether you think you can't do it or whether you don't feel like doing it yet. Just start. Practice this skill by unconditionally starting simply planned activities. Like for example, if you're planning to read a chapter of a book 30 minutes before you leave, then just do it without thinking about anything else.

To avoid stress related to cramming, you have to know

which activities will bring pressure and then you have to prioritize them over those that can merely bring pleasure. Whenever you are making a draft of your schedule, be sure to prioritize those activities that affect your work; they are the ones that will surely bring you pressure. However, you need to allot resting periods between your responsibilities, because if not, then you are just going to be very eager to finish your work so you can finally relax.

Relaxing is just as important as working, but with the current employment system these days, people are forced to have more time to work and less time to relax. Since you have so little time for relaxation, you must maximize the amount of tension released when you are relaxing. Ease yourself by diverting your attention from work to other things like listening to music, surfing the web, reading a good book, or chatting with your friends and colleagues - do anything as long as you find it enjoyable. If you fail to make the most out of your relaxation period, you are just going to end up looking for more time to relax and finding yourself panicking to finish your work.

Avoid Learning These Time Management Skills

When it comes to today's busy world, it seems that learning time management skills are a necessary asset to acquire in today's' world. Unfortunately, many people go about time management the wrong way and just end up getting burned out.

Are you learning these bad time management skills?

1. Giving everything equal importance to everything on your 'to do list'. By giving everything equal importance on your list, the important tasks suffer, and the unimportant tasks take up way too much of your precious time.

2. Making your 'to do list' too complicated. Many people feel the need to have fancy electronic organizers or the latest computer software help them organize their time. The best, easiest, and the fastest way is to keep a piece of paper in your pocket so you can capture ideas and notes at any time.

3. Doing unimportant tasks first. That advantage of your natural daily rhythm and do the most important tasks when you have the most energy. This time is likely in the morning, and not after lunch when you are starting to feel like taking a nap.

4. Being inconsistent. Some people start trying to learn time management skills and do okay, but then drop them and go back to their old ways. To be effective at time management you need to try and improve gradually every day.

5. Scheduling no time for yourself. Don't schedule your 'to do list' so you are running around all day. Make sure to schedule in some quiet time every day for yourself.

If you are learning these bad time management skills, it is time to stop. Learning about time management does not have to be hard. There is lots of great free information on the web today. Your goal should be a gradual improvement every day.

Time Management Skills - How They Help Students Achieve Success

Stories of grad students show a lot of courage in their ability to balance their academics with their huge list of important responsibilities:

This is a situation of a female student whose is faced with an intimidating task that may be given up easily by faint-hearted students. She is a grad student and is running a small scale business.

She is a mother of a child and lives in a room where the roommate has the worst of habits. As she goes on with her business, studies, mothering chores and household work, she is reminded of only one thing and time is very valuable.

Plenty of other such college students are balancing their responsibilities of completing their studies and struggling to make a livelihood. There are others who are toggling between extra-curricular activities and part-time jobs and still need to find time for their friends and families

For students of very high motivation, time is very precious. In order to accomplish their endeavors? They require proper management of time. Stress is brought upon students who have a very limiting and cramped day.

Failure to manage time properly results in stress. If you have failed in achieving certain tasks and goals, it would be followed by a vexed and stressful atmosphere.

The soul and body are severely affected by stress. Students lose their ability to accomplish their goals if stress invades the bodies of students.

Social skills and communication get affected badly. By this happening to us, we will be wasting a lot of time and money. Tuition in college is not very cheap. We should be completely sure that by committing ourselves to college and other responsibilities along with it, we should be ready to accomplish its demands; otherwise, it will lead to loss of time and money which could have been used in the future.

Grad students should not meander away from their crucial goals. If we do not accomplish what we were set to do, it will lead to highly disappointing failures.

We should not only get up early in the morning in order to meet our schedules in college but also need to meet the tuition fees payments and cope up to the expectations of your teachers and professors that they set.

A lot of students are still struggling because they do not have the courage to manage their time properly thereby making them very inflexible. There are general time management measures which allow you to put off your abilities, and helps you to find out your how far you can go.

Common student achieves their long-term task quickly by having the full-time course as part of the effort. This will be a perfect setting provided you have resources and time.

Find out the schedule of your presence needed for a particular course before enrolling. Be it a full-time or part-time job, consider what all is needed for it. Different time management techniques can be used depending on the nature of the job in order to schedule your studies.

If you have a job, time out your schedule in such a way that you cover all your activities, community colleges and universities give planners, clocks, and calendars in order to make up your schedule.

Negotiate with the administration to look into your

schedule. Classes around your job will be ideal for applying. Students with full-time jobs can take up online courses.

Not everybody is struggling with time. Highly prolific people manage their time efficiently and effectively handle things they set to do.

They know the knack of handling huge projects and finishing it without feeling stressed out. They look for balance and fulfillment of life and are making and accomplishing the most important goals.

We should know that a grad student requires being tough in body and soul. Time management skills are useless if it is not implemented in a correct strategy or method.

15: Finishing Your Thesis When You Believe You Can't

"How do I force myself to write when I can't stand looking at my thesis anymore?"

"I feel so guilty dragging my whole family down with this thesis writing, and I don't even know when I'll be done."

"No matter how much I do, there is always more. Will this EVER end?"

I have seen this cycle hundreds of times.

You start working on your thesis, pick up momentum, make progress, and then you hit a dead-end or open a can of worms.

Something that was supposed to take 2 days, takes 2 weeks or 1 month.

You feel guilty, maybe even ashamed.

"Why can't I just get this DONE? Everyone else is finishing up, what's wrong with me?"

This is depression kicking in...

You want to give up, but you are too far along to throw all this time and money away.

So you sit down and start working, and you feel like you are on track until (for one reason or another), you fall off the wagon.

This cycle can happen 10, 20 or 50 times.

The bad news is that each time you go through the cycle you get more frustrated, angry, bitter, resentful, and doubtful that will ever graduate.

You really start believing that you will never finish.

You can't even imagine what your life would be like without worrying about your thesis.

So, what's the good news?

The good news is that you WILL finish your research!!!

Once you recognize that you are in this cycle, you can break the habits that feed the cycle.

The only thing standing between you and finishing your thesis is your self-confidence (I talked about this in Part one of this ebook)

That's right: it's not the time or your thesis supervisor or your thesis committee.

When you have self-confidence and know beyond the shadow of any doubt that you have what it takes to finish your thesis, you can leap over any obstacle.
"But, how I can be confident when I am way behind?" you may be asking.

Here is something you may not have known:

Your self-confidence has nothing to do with how successful you are.

You would be surprised at how many over-achieving students, who have published extensively, have very little self-confidence.

They may think that they just got "lucky" when their papers were accepted, and they tremble at the thought of presenting their work at their next committee meeting.

On the other hand, there are students who have encountered every obstacle you can think of: dead-end projects, change of supervisor (if their previous supervisor moved), limited funding, but they are still confident that they will find a way to finish their thesis.

Who decides how confident you are?

You do.

Self-confidence is the antidote to the stress, anxiety, and writer's block that are holding you back now.

You can be confident no matter what.

Your self-confidence does not have to be shaken up after realizing that you messed up (again) or that you just lost 6 months of work.

Your self-confidence is your most important asset in grad school.

Without it, you will feel like a victim.

With it, you will become unstoppable, and you thesis will be DONE too.

4 Steps that Will Inevitably Lead to Finishing Your Thesis

1 - Get a crystal clear vision of what is expected from you

It is impossible to hit a target that you don't have, yet that is what many grad students try to do.

They plan on graduating in 6 or 12 months, but when I ask them what they need to do to finish their thesis they reply something like:

"I am not entirely sure…" or "I haven't brought it up with my committee…"

I get it.

I know how intimidating it can be to have the "talk" with your supervisor or stand in front of a committee.

But isn't the uncertainty of your future more intimidating?

How can you plan on finishing your thesis if you don't know what to do?

By definition, research is uncertain, and the requirements for your thesis will change as you collect and analyze data.

However, you can only adjust your trajectory when you are in motion.

You cannot make adjustments if you are standing still.

You need a vision, a starting point, that will help you to pick up momentum in your thesis.

2 - Rise and grind daily

I wish there was a nicer way of saying this, but there isn't.

There is no substitute for taking action daily.

If you working full-time or if you have a family, then working on your thesis daily may seem impossible.

It isn't.

I work with students who have multiple jobs, or several kids, yet they found a way to work on their thesis everyday.

They didn't necessarily work on it for hours, but they made a commitment to work on it at least a little bit every single day.

So, what is a "little bit" of time that you need to commit to your thesis daily?

It depends – the closer you are to finishing it, the more time you need to spend on it.

However, there is something magical about devoting at least 15 minutes a day to your thesis.

No matter how busy you are you can always find 15 minutes somewhere during your day.

It may be first thing in the morning, during your lunch hour at work, or in the evening (instead of TV or social media).

Why 15 minutes?

Fifteen minutes is long enough that if you are focused you can make measurable progress (write several paragraphs), but it is a short amount of time, so it seems doable every day.

Spending only 15 minutes a day on your thesis will probably not get you very far in the long run.

Most students with jobs or families spent at least 15 minutes a day on their thesis during the week, and then a longer block of time on the weekend.

So, what's the point of these short work sessions during the week (5 x 15 minutes is barely more than 1 hour)?

The point of daily commitment is continuity.

Continuity helps you to pick up where you left off, so that you don't have to spend 15-30 minutes trying to figure out what you are supposed to be doing.

When you spend at least a little time on your thesis every day, you get more creative, more ideas, and more insights that will help you to resolve problems that may have seemed impossible before.

3 - Focus on results, not "to-do"s

Do you feel like you are being pulled in 47 different directions each week?

Most grad students (and people in general), operate from a to-do list.

They write down all the work and non-related things that "should" do, but they give little thought to the tangible result they want to see.

When you let a "to-do" list run your life, you will always feel exhausted, and pla/ying catch up.

In fact, the more to-do's you cross off your list, the more to-do's you realize you need to get done.

As long as you live your life by a to-do list, you can't win, no matter how efficient you are.

It's time to try something new.

Instead of following a to-do list and cramming as much as possible into each day, write down what is the end result that you want.

For example, instead of writing in your calendar "Work on slides for committee meeting", write "Create an outstanding presentation for committee meeting to show them that my data is solid, and I am ready to move onto the next phase of my research".

Then, you can list the actions necessary to achieve that result.

An action plan with a well-defined goal for finishing your thesis is much more motivating than a random list of chores.

With a results-oriented action plan you will be able to prioritize better and take the actions that will help you to make the most progress in your thesis.

After all, you don't want to become a slave to your to-list – you just want a finished your thesis!

4 - Soak up the energy you need from a support group

The number one complaint of grad students is that they feel isolated and lost their motivation to do work.

In grad school, there are support groups in the form of study groups, office hours, and the residential community.

In graduate school, many students do not have any type of support.

First-year students usually start out with enthusiasm, but due to lack of accountability they lose track of time and fall behind on their milestones.

In contrast, the students who did join a support group

thought that being part of a community was one of the best ways to keep themselves motivated.

There is no shame in getting support, whether it is academic or emotional support to help you focus on finishing your thesis.

Don't take my word for it.

The #1 advice from PhDs for graduate students for finishing your thesis is to join a support group.

The more people you "worry" with, the more perspectives you get and the smaller your problems seem.

When you live in your own head, you can blow a minor issue out of proportion.

Suddenly, taking off two days from work because you didn't feel well may seem like a huge setback until you hear from others that what you are going through is normal for a graduate student.

There will be times when you feel so burnt out that you will not want to work for weeks.

Or, you may start doubting the point of grad school when you don't know what you'll do afterwards.

Without a context, these situations can rob you of your self-confidence and your motivation.

How could you be motivated when you identify yourself as "lazy" and think there is no point in finishing your thesis anyway?

You can sort out these sticky situations by sharing with others, especially graduate students who are going through similar experiences, and feel better about your experience in school, college and university.

So if you are wondering how to get motivated to write a thesis when you would rather do anything else, look no further than support from other graduate students.

Just knowing that you are not the only one going through these tribulations can already take most of the pressure off that has been keeping you from being motivated to work on your thesis.

Make a commitment to yourself to get the support you need, because you have what is it takes to finish your thesis.

FINAL NOTE

You're not being selfish or a burden to ask someone to take you to the hospital if you break your leg. Likewise, you're not being selfish to ask someone to help you with a mental illness. If they can't help you themselves, maybe they can help you to get in contact with a local therapist or local team at your school, college or university. It's not shameful. It's necessary.

You also need to be more open to going out with those around you. If you're invited, say yes! Expand your support group by making friends.

If you're struggling with maintaining mental health while researching, please know that you're not alone. Try to seek help.

The place you're in is well worth exploring. It is a privilege to go to a school, college or university, and you should be able to enjoy it. Equip yourself with the people and tools you need to have the best trip possible.

Keep the hard work up, stay motivated and think positive. You have come across a long way to be here, and you are not far from reaching your goals.

"The price of success is hard work, dedication to the job at hand, and the determination that whether we win or lose, we have applied the best of ourselves to the task at hand"
– Vince Lombardi.

RESOURCES:

- Everyday Health: www.everydayhealth.com
- National Institue of Mental Health: www.nimh.nih.gov
- Finish Your Thesis: www.finishyourthesis.com
- National Health Services: www.nhs.net
- Mind for better mental health: www.mind.org.uk
- OncoNano Research Group

Acknowledgements

First, I would like to thank my family for the fantastic support.

I would like to thank Professor Mehmet Dorak for his incredible support and motivation for keeping me inspired during his postgraduate statistics lectures.

A debt of gratitude is also owed to Professor Ivan Roitt and Professor Richard Bayford for being amazing PhD supervisors and keeping me motivated throughout the last few years.

Last but not least, I would like to thank the editors of this book Rahmanullah Hayat and Sadiya Nazmeen Ali for fantastic work.

Thank you Professor Mehmet Dorak for telling me to write down the quote below in my statistics lecture notebook. "Strive for progress, not perfection" - Vince Lombardi.

About the Author

Fahimullah Hayat is a final year PhD student in antibiotics resistance and biophysics research, Fahimullah Hayat set up OncoNano Research Group in his university to help people with self-esteem, anxiety, stress, assertiveness and related difficulties. From many years Fahimullah Hayat is working with many different organisations such as retailers, charity services, emergency services and with other organisations.

Fahimullah Hayat is keen in developing programs and initiatives to help students to tackle any issues within their study places. Fahimullah Hayat is further working on developing a multidisciplinary model within the education centres where student barriers can be self-analysed and assessed.

Available worldwide from Amazon
and all good bookstores

———————

www.mtp.agency

www.facebook.com/mtp.agency

@mtp_agency

www.ingramcontent.com/pod-product-compliance
Lightning Source LLC
LaVergne TN
LVHW091548060526
838200LV00036B/751